PSYCHOSOCIAL ASSESSMENT

A Pocket Guide for Data Collection

AF863418

Lois Grey Long, R.N., M.S.
Assistant Professor Emeritus
School of Nursing
The University of Texas
Health Science Center at San Antonio
San Antonio, Texas

Patricia Grant Higgins, R.N., M.S., Ph.D.
Assistant Professor
College of Nursing
The University of New Mexico
Albuquerque, New Mexico

Debra Brady, R.N., M.N.Ed.
Nursing Education Consultant
New Mexico State Board of Nursing
Albuquerque, New Mexico

APPLETON & LANGE
Norwalk, Connecticut/San Mateo, California

0-8385-8030-0

Notice: The author(s) and publisher of this volume have taken care that the information and recommendations contained herein are accurate and compatible with the standards generally accepted at the time of publication.

Copyright © 1988 by Appleton & Lange
A Publishing Division of Prentice Hall

All rights reserved. This book, or any parts thereof, may not be used or reproduced in any manner without written permission. For information, address Appleton & Lange, 25 Van Zant Street, East Norwalk, Connecticut 06855.

88 89 90 91 92 / 10 9 8 7 6 5 4 3 2 1

Prentice-Hall of Australia, Pty. Ltd., Sydney
Prentice-Hall Canada, Inc.
Prentice-Hall Hispanoamericana, S.A., Mexico
Prentice-Hall of India Private Limited, New Delhi
Prentice-Hall International (UK) Limited, London
Prentice-Hall of Japan, Inc., Tokyo
Prentice-Hall of Southeast Asia (Pte.) Ltd., Singapore
Whitehall Books Ltd., Wellington, New Zealand
Editora Prentice-Hall do Brasil Ltda., Rio de Janeiro

Library of Congress Cataloging-in-Publication Data

Long, Lois Grey.
Psychosocial assessment.

1. Medical history taking. 2. Nursing. I. Higgins, Patricia Grant. II. Brady, Debra. III. Title.
RT48.5.L66 1987 610.73 87-15914
ISBN 0-8385-8030-0

Production Editor: Sandra Swindler
Designer: M. Chandler Martylewski
Cover: Kathleen Peters

PRINTED IN THE UNITED STATES OF AMERICA

To our families, who provide the ongoing special support that makes this vast a project possible.

CONTENTS

PREFACE

An accurate assessment of the client provides a solid foundation on which to base nursing diagnosis, planning, intervention and evaluation—the other steps of nursing process. No phase of this process stands alone and the nurse will find that as the client is assessed, intervention through the use of therapeutic communication skills may be necessary. This can assist the client in problem solving.

This text enables the reader to obtain an accurate psychosocial assessment of the client by pulling together comprehensive psychosocial assessment information which exists only in pieces throughout various journals and books. Psychosocial assessment is addressed in concise units that begin by describing the area of concern and follow with a list of questions touching on important points within the area. After the preliminary questions follow modifications for individuals with specific needs: i.e., older adult, expectant parent, newborn, infant, child, and adolescent.

Our goal is to enable the reader to holistically assess the psychosocial needs of the client, which in turn will promote more complete and appropriate care. This book is meant to be more than a group of questions. It is important that the student using this book recognizes that no client can accurately be assessed merely by asking a series of questions. The nurse must be sensitive to verbal cues indicating that an area should be assessed in more detail. We remind the reader that the nurse assessing the client from the psychosocial dimension obtains information that is highly personal. The nurse must maintain the confidentiality of this information so that a trusting and therapeutic relationship develops between the nurse and the client as a basis for productive intervention. Note that no data base is ever complete. It will always be necessary for the nurse to work with the information already obtained and to continue to gather data with each client visit.

We caution that the nurse also needs to keep in mind that this book offers guidelines for the assessment of the psychosocial dimension only. To assess the client holistically the nurse will need to incorporate assessment of other dimensions into the care of the client.

ACKNOWLEDGMENTS

We acknowledge the assistance of many people in making this book possible. First, our thanks go to Carma Trujillo, who typed the initial proposal when it was truly a rough draft, and thus a difficult task. Our appreciation also to Erma Pohl, Eleanor DeHahn and Peggy Evilsizer, typists who each helped with refinements as the manuscript went through the stages of development.

Molding and guidance was offered by our reviewers and we wish to express appreciation for the suggestions and contributions from Ann Doyle, R.N., M.S.N., City College, Shirley Hoeman, M.S.N., Nola Pender, R.N., Ph.D., Northern Illinois University, JoAnne Ryan, R.N., Ph.D., University of Delaware, and Susan Stevens, R.N., D.S.N., University of South Carolina.

Our thanks to Dorothy Roehr, R.N., B.S.N., M.L.A., for her suggestions, guidance, and proofreading as we developed the manuscript.

Above all, without the assistance, diplomacy, and problem-solving skills of our editor, Marion Kalstein-Welch, this book would not have been possible.

Our thanks to all.

Lois
Pat
Deb

INTRODUCTION

This book is the cumulative result of our efforts to incorporate psychosocial assessment skills into nursing care planning, which frequently is dominated by physical assessment with occasional related psychosocial components. We are specialists in gerontological nursing, maternal–newborn nursing, health education, and medical–surgical nursing. The diversity of our backgrounds, preparations, and approaches to health care led us to develop these guidelines on psychosocial assessment, which are as comprehensive as possible.

Psychosocial assessment information is available in the literature; however, in our age of specialization, it is widely scattered in textbooks and journals in the different specialty areas in nursing and allied health professions. This book is a composite of assessment guidelines applicable across the life-span accumulated from the literature of nursing and the psychosocial sciences. It is presented in a concise format for ease in reference. The use of this book along with any of the excellent physical assessment texts currently available will provide parameters for obtaining a broader and more complete picture of the client's level of functioning.

This book is written with the baccalaureate nursing student in mind, but should be helpful to other nursing students as well. In each of the psychosocial concepts selected, we have tried to indicate as thoroughly as possible the kinds of concepts that are important to a holistic assessment in the data-gathering step of the nursing process. It is important to recognize that no data base is ever complete because the client and the environment are ever changing. It is always necessary to work with the information at hand and continue to expand the data base as it relates to the individual's development throughout the life-span.

The psychosocial assessment questions in this book are presented in columnar format. The adult material appears first, followed by questions for the older adult, the expectant parent, and newborn. Assessment questions for the infant/child/adolescent are grouped together last.

HOW TO USE THIS BOOK

The first part provides the reader with a review of the theoretical foundations necessary to focus on psychosocial health assessment. Part 2 consists of 13 units that have been designed to provide guidance in obtaining a relatively complete psychosocial assessment. To maintain the concept of holism, data should be added to each unit of the psychosocial assessment data base as one has additional contact with the client.

The question format is designed so that regardless of the client's age, questions from the adult column should usually be selected and asked first. When this procedure is completed, depending on the age of the client, appropriate questions from the client's age column should be asked. For example, the client is Mrs. X, age 80, who is having difficulty sleeping. The collection of information should begin with the adult column of the demographic section. To this the interviewer would add demographic information questions from the older adult column. The interviewer would then turn to the unit on sleep and select appropriate questions from the adult column, supplementing these with questions from the older adult column in the sleep unit. Each of the 13 units in this book is designed to be used in approximately this same manner.

To use this book properly the student must possess an understanding of interviewing skills. If not, review of this topic may be necessary. It is important to recognize that only portions of this psychosocial data can be gathered in any one client encounter. Each time there is a client meeting or contact, more data is gathered to expand the data base, thus increasing the potential effectiveness of nursing care planning. If the student finds a need to assess additional portions of the client's life-style or activities, the bibliographical references throughout the book can be used to locate more specific guidelines to assist with this task.

Psychosocial assessment is part of the first phase of the nursing process. After data are gathered from the physical and psychosocial dimensions the nursing process should be continued, using this data to plan, intervene, and evaluate the client's needs and progress.

GUIDELINES FOR PSYCHOSOCIAL ASSESSMENT

The Value of Psychosocial Assessment

Psychosocial data collection is important because this assessment is part of the basis of the entire nursing process. If the psychosocial data are complete and accurate, the planning will be appropriate. Psychosocial assessment is the gathering of data about emotional, behavioral, mental, environmental, and interactional processes. Collection of new data must also include integration of the information with that already existing and with the physical assessment data to obtain as complete a profile of the individual as possible. Data are gathered by the nurse in an effort to identify the individual's past and current level of functioning. The biophysical factors interact reciprocally with the psychosocial factors throughout the life cycle. The interplay among these factors leads to a higher level of individual functioning, organizing, and adapting as the client progresses across the life-span.

The psychosocial assessment is part of the responsibility of every nurse and should be done at every client encounter as part of a comprehensive, ongoing assessment. As psychosocial assessment skills are developed by the nurse and used along with the physical assessment, the gap that frequently exists in data collection will be bridged so that clients may be treated more efficiently, correctly, successfully, and holistically.

Psychosocial assessment is much more than a series of questions. It is the process of interacting with the client in many different situations to evaluate the level of psychosocial functioning. The assessment requires multiple observations of the client and his or her lifestyle for it to be as complete as possible.

I

CONCEPTUAL FRAMEWORK

Too often, nurses limit their view of the client to the disease process involved and focus on the physical aspects of the patient's care. Care givers' efforts are directed toward the fractured femur or the pregnant abdomen without adequate attention to the person attached to the physical problem. The emphasis in nursing literature is on the medical model and physical assessment. The psychosocial components of patient assessment are fragmented, frequently by specialty areas. For example, the nurse may have difficulty assessing the person with a fracture who also has a nutrition problem. Therefore, we have included three concepts to bridge the gap between physical and psychosocial assessment: holism, developmental theory, and nursing process (Fig. 1).

CONCEPTUAL MODEL FOR PSYCHOSOCIAL ASSESSMENT

We believe that the client should be viewed as a total person, a holistic view incorporating the physical, mental, emotional, spiritual, and social dimensions, with each of these aspects interacting to form the unique individual. In the model (Fig. 1) on which this book is based, the life cycle begins with the adult because adults make up the largest portion of the population. One then moves from the adult years into the older years. The adult and older adult support the individuals who begin the cycle of the next generation, with the expectant parent and newborn followed by the infant/child/adolescent years.

As one proceeds through the life cycle, emphasis for psychoso-

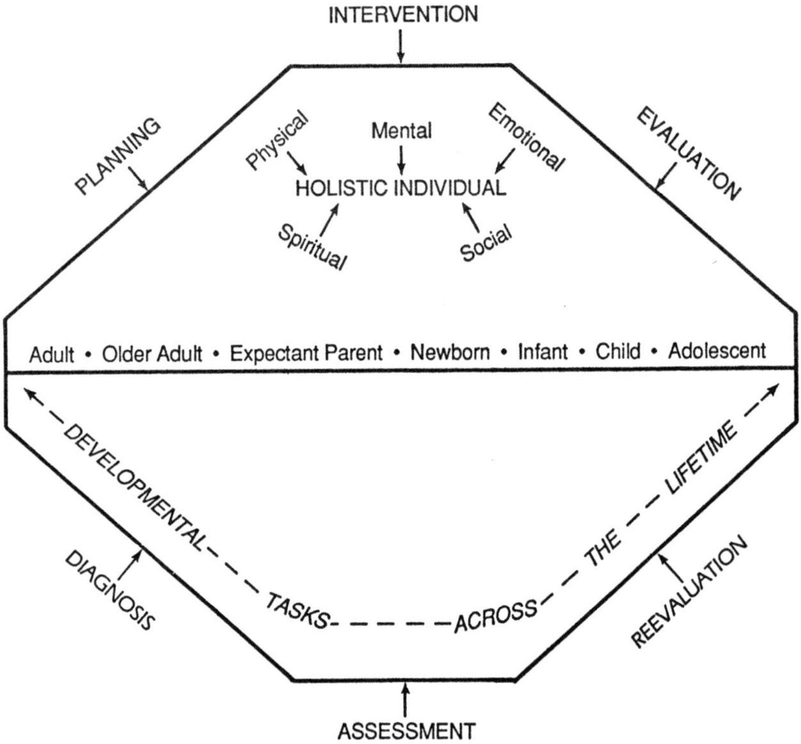

Figure 1. The conceptual framework for psychosocial assessment.

cial assessment changes. For example, during the adolescent years the major emphasis is on social issues and physical changes. The adult questions focus less on the physical aspects and more on dimensions such as career and family, whereas the older adult may concentrate on adaptation to aging changes and relative state of health.

The nursing process is the tool used by nurses to assess, plan, implement, and evaluate the holistic care for the client. Thus, the first step in the nursing process is the holistic assessment. Both physical and psychosocial assessments should be conducted with the individual and/or family focusing on various points along the continuum of the life-span.

Each individual should be assessed as a total person regardless of the presenting problems. For example, Mr. Jones, a security guard at the university, has fractured his femur. A typical nursing assessment would focus primarily on the physical problem, with less thought given to this adult as a total person. Mr. Jones may be more concerned about how he will support his wife and two children than in learning how to walk with crutches. A psychosocial assessment of this client would identify other needs beyond the physical and allow the nurse to formulate a more complete plan of care. The concepts of holism, developmental theory and nursing process are the keys to psychosocial assessment and are expanded further. Physical examination, including the mental status evaluation, is adequately described and discussed in the literature. The effort here is to address the psychosocial components of holism.

HOLISM

The concept of holism is closely related to health. Both words are derived from the same Anglo-Saxon root, *hol*, which can mean whole, to heal, sound, or happy. D. C. Phillips (1976) identified several points relating to holism:

1. The whole is more than the sum of its parts.
2. The whole determines the nature of its parts.
3. The parts cannot be understood if considered in isolation from the whole.
4. The parts are dynamically interrelated or interdependent.

The person has traditionally been viewed piecemeal, in terms of the physical, mental, emotional, social, and spiritual dimensions. Frequently one dimension is emphasized more than others, depending on the educational preparation of the professional person doing the evaluation. When this division occurs, the needs of the client are often not fully understood. Rarely does a physical problem, such as a baby with colic or an older adult with vision problems, not also impact other dimensions of the person's life. Only when the nurse assesses the whole person and not just the problem area will a complete plan of care be possible.

No two individuals are alike. Each person is a unique combination of physical, mental, emotional, social and spiritual aspects. The life-style that one chooses and develops is based upon knowledge, values, culture, attitudes, motivation and behavior. In addition to assessing the many facets of the individual, the nurse must approach each aspect of assessment with a recognition of the uniqueness of the person. The approach that the nurse uses with an adult may not be effective when assessing the child. With the child, the nurse can be creative in her or his interviewing techniques by incorporating questions into a game. For example, the perception of interpersonal relationships with the family may be determined by asking the child to draw a picture of the family.

The uniqueness of an individual consists of many complex aspects that change throughout the growth and development process. These changes can vary from day to day and week to week. Therefore, the nurse must develop a unique relationship with each client to incorporate the points developed by Phillips and thus practice holistic nursing. Also, holistic nursing practice requires an understanding of health and wellness. Health is usually defined in a positive sense. Halbert L. Dunn defined health as:

> . . . an integrated method of functioning which is oriented toward maximizing the potential of which the individual is capable, within the environment where he is functioning.

Dunn stated that health or wellness was not fixed but an ongoing process toward an even higher potential of functioning. He developed the directional concept of "high-level wellness" (Dunn, 1961).

Don Ardell considered the concepts of wellness, prevention, and adaptation and defined high-level wellness as a:

> . . . lifestyle-focused approach which you design for the purpose of pursuing the highest level of health within your capability. A wellness lifestyle is dynamic or ever-changing as you evolve throughout life. It is an integrated lifestyle in that you incorporate some approach or aspect of each wellness dimension (self-responsibility, nutritional awareness, stress management, physical fitness, and environmental sensitivity). (Ardell, 1977)

Definitions of holism and health have changed over time, along with our beliefs and theories about wellness and illness. The same is true for assessment. By using psychosocial assessment along with physical assessment, one is able to take a holistic view of the client.

The goal of holistic nursing is to maintain human integrity (Yura & Walsh, 1983). When the nurse assimilates the interrelationships of the 12 constructs (culture, environmental safety, exercise, leisure activities, interpersonal relationships, medications, emotional health, nutrition, sexuality, sleep, spirituality, substance use) the client's holistic integrity is preserved. Adequate assessment in each of these areas is required so that plans and interventions can be proposed to maintain the client's health and wellness along the life continuum.

To help the individual maintain health and meet personal needs at various points in the life cycle, the nurse makes use of diverse knowledge and skills. By understanding and applying concepts from such related disciplines as sociology, psychology and human relations along with those of nursing, the nurse incorporates the concept of holism into client care. Skill in using the nursing process will increase the nurse's ability to view the client holistically.

DEVELOPMENTAL THEORY AND TASKS

When the nurse assesses a person from a holistic point of view, it is necessary to consider developmental theory and specific developmental tasks applicable to that individual. The discussion of developmental theory here is brief because most students have had courses in growth and development and studied various developmental theories prerequisite to entering a baccaulaureate nursing program.

Developmental tasks are so named because as they are sequentially completed, they lead to ever higher levels of organization and adaptation. Tasks in one life stage generally must be successfully completed to build a solid foundation for the next set of tasks. Theorists usually begin their life-cycle discussion with infancy and suggest a series of developmental tasks to be completed by the person across the life-span. In this book, however, the adult is presented first because the majority of our population is in the adult years. We have attempted to assemble the most complete set of guidelines for psychosocial assessment for the adult and then have built on this foundation for the other age-groups. The adult years are divided into two groups, young adulthood (the ages between 20 and 40) and the middle years (those from age 40 to 60). The young adult's developmental tasks include the selection of an occupation; finding a mate and learning to live within the relationship; making decisions about having and rearing children; managing a home; and establishing an adult relationship with parents. Developmental tasks for the middle adult include achieving civic and social responsibility and maintaining the economic basis for the standard of living. Within the middle adult years there is a need to evaluate aspirations, abandon unreachable goals and reorder remaining priorities toward more achievable outcomes. Middle adult years may bring personal losses in the form of divorce and the death of parents and some contemporaries, requiring substantial adaptation. Another developmental task for this age-group is the development of leisure-time activities and acceptance of the physiological changes that may occur with progression through the adult years.

The years beyond this period are those of the older adult or later maturity. Developmental tasks at this age include the ongoing adjustment to decreasing physical strength and health, as well as to retirement and often to reduced income as a result of no longer being employed. The deaths of peers, relatives, and friends continue and eventually will include one's spouse. Circumstances may force changes in living arrangements. Developmental tasks include many adjustments to these differing circumstances and maintenance of a life-style as active as possible by replacing an occupation with other interests. There are times that there is reorganization of needs and priorities, but the developmental process continues throughout human life in a sequence that is generally predictable and has been studied enough to be fairly well defined.

The adult age-groups give rise to the beginning of another generation, which starts with the expectant parents. Developmental tasks for the expectant parent vary from those of the adult principally in the preparation for and the bearing of children. According to Duvall, tasks for the group include planning for housing and financial support for the couple and then the new baby. The couple must incorporate specific knowledge and activities having to do with pregnancy, birth, and parenthood into the relationship. This period also includes the assigning of tasks within the family and adapting to relationships with relatives and friends (Duvall, 1977).

Successful completion of the developmental tasks for newly married couples facilitates successful accomplishment of the parental role and the developmental tasks of infancy and toddlerhood, the period from birth to age three. Tasks for this age-group include learning to walk, talk, control elimination and distinguish between right and wrong. The child's bond with the mother is the first significant relationship in life. The child begins some physical separation from the parents during the second six months by crawling, followed by standing and then walking at about one year of age. The child must establish a personal identity, and an important task for this age is to detach from the mother.

The remaining years until age 20 are usually divided between early childhood years (age 3 to 6), childhood (age 6 to puberty), and adolescence (puberty to age 20). During the early childhood years the child has growing interest in father, siblings, family relationships, and eventually friends. During the childhood years, friends become more important as peers and companions. The child must learn to function within parental and societal rules and cope with new situations. Anger and frustration must be vented appropriately. As the child forms a conscience and increases the ability to express needs and ideas, inner control of behavior develops. These processes permit the child to increase participation in activities outside the home, including sports and hobbies. The adolescent years include the physical changes to an adult body and developmental tasks of achieving emotional independence from parents, learning appropriate masculine or feminine roles, accepting one's physical changes, and finding outlets for new sexual feelings that are acceptable to family and society. The adolescent must select and begin preparation for an occupation and continue developing socially responsible behavior.

The nurse needs to recognize that most persons make ongoing conscious and subconscious efforts to satisfactorily accomplish developmental tasks. Assessing the level of achievement of appropriate developmental tasks for the client is an important part of planning holistic care for the total person.

NURSING PROCESS

The nursing process is the method by which nurses solve problems. It is the essence of nursing, which allows all nurses to share a common language. The process is applicable in any setting because it is adaptable and flexible. Therefore, it is basic to providing holistic nursing care for clients at each developmental level across the life-span.

The nursing process consists of four phases: assessment, planning, implementation, and evaluation. Each of these phases is dependent upon the other; none stands alone. There are no distinct lines separating one unit from the other. It is an orderly, systematic manner of determining the client's problems, making plans to solve them, initiating the plan or assigning others to implement it, and evaluating the extent to which the plan was effective in resolving the problems identified (Yura & Walsh, 1983).

Four components essential to an accurate, successful use of the nursing process are that it be planned, client-, family-, or community-focused, problem-oriented, and goal-directed. A plan implies a conscious, deliberate, and systematic effort to attain a goal. Without a plan chaos ensues because all aspects of the problem and solutions have not been considered. If the client is not included in determining the role he or she will play in the process, it is likely that client goals could be different from those of the nurse, leading to difficulty in achieving outcomes within the plan.

To successfully use the nursing process, the nurse must acquire several skills. These are intellectual or problem-solving skills, interpersonal or communication skills, and technical or physical assessment skills. The foundation for these skills is provided in the basic nursing program, and they are integrated and refined with experience over time.

Factors inherent in developing and refining these skills include an understanding of one's own strengths, limitations, patterns of response, views, and values. This self-awareness will help the nurse to accept the client as a unique, holistic individual. Developing this self-awareness can be aided by understanding some basic principles of behavior that affect the interaction process. Assumptions about behavior to keep in mind when using the nursing process include:

1. A person's response to a stimulus equals the behavior. All behavior has covert and overt aspects. Thoughts, feelings,

and motivations constitute the covert aspect, whereas actions and verbalizations make up the overt aspect.
2. Behavior is governed by the amount of energy the person has available at any given time. Individuals differ in their energy potential because of many factors including age, sex, food intake, basal metabolic rate, condition of the atmosphere and the number of stresses with which the person must cope in any given time period.
3. All behavior has a purpose even though it may not always be obvious.
4. The person's response to a situation is the best of which he or she is capable at that time.
5. The perception of the person about what is happening is more important than what is actually happening or another person's interpretation of what is happening.
6. Moving forward is a potential for all people.

It is important that the nurse recognize behavioral factors that may be operating in the client, the nurse, or both of them, because these behaviors have a profound influence upon interaction (Brown & Fowler, 1971).

Prepared with the basic skills and an understanding of behavior and interaction, the nurse is now ready to set the stage upon which the nursing process will be carried out. In order to do this the nurse uses interpersonal skills to establish a trust with the client, define the role she or he will play in the client's care, allow the client an opportunity to voice fears and ask questions, and establish a positive environment in which the process can be carried out. Effective interpersonal communication skills are essential to a holistic assessment, and these skills should be reviewed as necessary. Taking the time and care to establish a therapeutic relationship will contribute much to the success of the process.

Any discussion of the nursing process is not complete without a definition of each phase of the process. Purposeful, organized, and logical collection of data and then the assignment of meaning to those data is the first phase of the process. These are two very distinct stages of the assessment phase. Factual data must be collected and analyzed separately to guard against assignment of meaning or conclusions based upon insufficient evidence.

The assessment phase begins with the collection of subjective and objective data. Subjective data are the client's reported experience of what he or she sees, hears, feels, or thinks. Objective data, on the other hand, are data that can be observed or measured by the nurse. These data should be verified or validated with the client to make sure they are accurate.

Data collection is ongoing rather than static, and the nurse gathers data at every client contact. The purpose of collecting this data is to determine the problems that the client is experiencing. Once the data are collected, the nurse then moves into the second stage of this phase, assignment of meaning to the data, problem identification, or making a nursing diagnosis. At this point the information collected is compared to a standard or norm to determine the client's problems and also his or her resources. Several categories of problems are identified by the nurse while analyzing data. These include actual, potential, or resolved. Actual problems are those that are occurring at the present time. A problem that the client has a high risk of developing, if something is not done to prevent it, is termed a potential problem. Resolved problems are those problems that caused significant difficulties in the past and may cause difficulty in the future. Resources are the available strengths or means of support a client has to overcome problems.

Once the problems have been identified, the nurse moves to the second phase of the process called planning. During this phase the nurse, along with the client, assigns priorities to the problems so that the most important ones can be addressed first. Goals are then determined. These are statements that indicate desired outcomes if the problem is resolved. The goals may be short- or long-term in nature. A series of short-term goals may eventually lead to the achievement of a long-term goal. Goals are stated in measurable terms so that the outcome of the process can be evaluated.

After the goals are determined, a plan of intervention is developed, based on the holistic assessment. In the development of a plan of intervention, many strategies may be considered. From this pool of ideas, appropriate interventions are then selected, considering the following factors, which determine whether or not the intervention will be successful.

1. Are the interventions based on a holistic assessment?
2. Does the intervention have a sound basis in theory?

3. Is the intervention compatible with the client's beliefs?
4. Are there resources available to accomplish the intervention?
5. Do the interventions include the client's resources?

In addition to answering these questions, the nurse will also need to evaluate each intervention for risks and side effects before incorporating it into the plan of care. The purpose of the nursing intervention is to achieve the goal and solve the problem.

Putting the plan into action, or implementation, is the third phase of the process. Depending upon the circumstances, the nurse may implement the plan by using any one of several methods. These include personally caring for the client; delegating care to others; referring the client to a specialist; and coordinating the activities of those persons interacting with the client.

Evaluation is the final phase of the process. At this time, the nurse once again collects subjective and objective data and compares them with the goal to determine if the goal has been accomplished The actual outcome of the nursing care is judged to determine the success of the nursing intervention. Some problems may be resolved, whereas others are not, and the nurse would then gather more data, change the plan, implement new strategies, and evaluate the outcome again; thus the cycle is repeated.

SUMMARY

A conceptual framework for psychosocial assessment has been proposed. The three major areas that have been discussed are:

1. The principles incorporated within holism to view the individual as a complex, whole, dynamic being, all of whose dimensions are interrelated
2. The developmental process of the individual and the unique tasks as one advances through the life-span
3. The nursing process as a problem-solving approach using physical and psychosocial assessment

Because we believe that people are holistic individuals, not just the sum of their component parts, we think that the nursing process should focus on the whole client. In recent years our profession has focused on the physical component of health assessment, sometimes to the exclusion of the psychological, environmental, and sociocultural aspects. The overall goal of the nurse for the client as a person is a highest-attainable level of wellness within the context of the individual physical, mental, emotional, social, and spiritual assessment. The life process is dynamic in nature and is on a continuum. The nurse who believes in and uses this conceptual framework is indeed practicing holistic nursing.

REFERENCES

Ardell, D. B. *High-level wellness.* Emmaus, Pa.: Rodale Press, 1977, p. 65.

Brown, M., & Fowler, G. *Psycho-dynamic nursing.* Philadelphia: Saunders, 1971, pp. 21–23.

Dunn, H. L. *High-level wellness.* Arlington, Va.: R. W. Beatty, 1961, pp. 5–6.

Duvall, E. M. *Marriage and family development.* Philadelphia: Lippincott, 1977, pp. 195–203.

Phillips, D. C. *Holistic thought in social science.* Stanford, Calif.: Stanford University Press, 1976, p. 6.

Yura, H., & Walsh, M. B. *The nursing process* (4th ed.). Norwalk, Conn.: Appleton-Century-Crofts, 1983, p. 307.

BIBLIOGRAPHY

Atkinson, D., & Murray, M. E. *Understanding the nursing process.* New York: Macmillan, 1983.

Blatner, B. *Holistic nursing.* Englewood Cliffs, N.J.: Prentice-Hall, 1981.

Brunner, L., & Suddarth, D. *Textbook of medical–surgical nursing.* Philadelphia: Lippincott, 1980.

Dubos, R. *Man-adapting.* New Haven, Conn.: Yale University Press, 1965.

Epstein, C. *The nurse leader: Philosophy and practice.* Reston, Va.: Reston Publishing, 1982.

Erikson, E. H. *Childhood and society.* New York: Norton, 1964.

Fields, W., & McGinn-Campbell, K. *Introduction to health assessment.* Reston, Va.: Reston Publishing, 1983.

Havighurst, R. J. *Human development and education.* New York: Longman, Green, 1953.

La Monica, L. *The nursing process: A humanistic approach.* Menlo Park, Calif.: Addison-Wesley, 1979.

Lewis, S., & Collier, I. *Medical–surgical nursing: Assessment and management of clinical problems.* New York: McGraw-Hill, 1983.
Marriner, A. *The nursing process: A scientific approach to nursing care.* St. Louis: Mosby, 1983.
Mayers, M. G. *A systematic approach to the nursing care plan* (3rd ed.). Norwalk, Conn.: Appleton-Century-Crofts, 1983.
Phipps, W., Long, B., & Woods, N. *Medical–surgical nursing concepts and clinical practice.* St. Louis: Mosby, 1983.
Piaget, J. *The origins of intelligence in children.* (M. Cook, trans.) New York: Norton, 1963.
Thompson, J., & Bowers, A. *Clinical manual of health assessment.* St. Louis: Mosby, 1980.
Yura, H., & Walsh, M. *The nursing process* (4th ed.). Norwalk, Conn.: Appleton-Century-Crofts, 1983.

II

GUIDELINES FOR PSYCHOSOCIAL ASSESSMENT

This part of the text is composed of 13 units:

1. Demographic Information
2. Culture
3. Environmental Safety
4. Exercise
5. Leisure Activities
6. Nutrition
7. Sleep
8. Emotional Health
9. Spirituality
10. Interpersonal Relationships
11. Sexuality
12. Medications
13. Substance Use

Each unit is introduced by a discussion and a definition of the construct, viewed developmentally across the life-span. The psychosocial assessment questions covered in this book are presented beginning with the adult, followed by the older adult, the expectant parent, the newborn, and finally the infant/child/adolescent.

UNIT 1

Demographic Information

INTRODUCTION

The starting point for psychosocial assessment is the gathering of the identifying or demographic data, which include information on the client's sex, religion, language, birth, family, marital status, education, occupation, income, and residence. An evaluation of the consistency of the responses from the client is important because it will allow the nurse to make some judgments about the client's reliability as an informant. Should the informant appear to be unreliable, it may be necessary for the nurse to seek the needed information from the client's family or friends or care givers.

Provided within this unit is a demographic data base for the adult. To use this data base for the older adult client, simply gather the additional data included in the older adult column. When assessing the infant, child, or adolescent client, collect the additional information included in those columns and delete any duplicated information in the adult column.

QUESTIONNAIRE

ADULT

What is your:

Full name?

Nickname or preferred first name?

Address?

Telephone number (residence and work)?

Date of birth?

Birthplace?

Citizenship or immigration status?

Ethnic background?

Primary language?

Other languages?

Place in the family?

Religion?

Marital status?

What is your spouse's or partner's:

Name?

Date of birth?

Religion?

Place of birth, ethnic background?

What was your courtship duration?

Date of marriage or when you began living together?

What are your children's names?

What are their sex and ages?

What is their city and state of residence?

If deceased, give date and cause (for women include miscarriages, stillbirths).

Are your parents living?

Have there been other marriages or partnerships?

What is your educational background?

How many years of school have you completed?

What is your occupation, place of employment, or are you self-employed?

Average number of hours worked per day and days per week?

Work interests, second occupation or profession?

What were the last three jobs and duration of employment?

If not currently employed, would you like to be?

Have you been in the military service; if so, branch, years, rank?

What are your sources of income or economic assistance? (Consider employment, social security, supplemental security income, veteran or disability benefits, family or public assistance, insurance payments, annuities, savings, investments, alimony, child support, food stamps.)

What is your health care insurance coverage? (Consider medicaid [number], employer-paid medical and dental.)

Means of transportation to health care facility?

Modifications for the Older Adult

Have you moved since retirement and if so, from where?

Are your living arrangements different since retirement and if so, how?

Is your spouse living? If not, date of death?

Who is to be contacted first in case of emergency? (Consider child or responsible party.)

When did you retire (date)?

What was your age at the time?

Was it voluntary, welcome, compulsory, forced?

Did you have preretirement preparation, counseling?

Have you worked since retirement?

What are your retirement sources of income? (Consider private, federal, railroad, or military pension; IRA; self-employed plan, [SEP].)

What is your medicare number?

Modifications for the Expectant Parent

Do you feel your housing is adequate for your expanded family?

Do you have a room designated and furnished as a nursery?

Modifications for the Newborn

Have you obtained a copy of the new baby's legal birth certificate?

Did the birth occur in home, hospital, birthing center?

Modifications for the Infant/Child/Adolescent

What is your parent or guardian's name?

In case of divorce or separation of parents, do you live with the parent of your choice?

Do you see the other parent as often as you would like?

What is your present grade in school?

Do you have an allowance?

UNIT 2
Culture

INTRODUCTION

A culture is composed of individuals who are born to or choose to share a set of learned values, beliefs, practices, and information. A cultural group incorporates experiences from the past, which influence the present and the traditions as passed to future generations. Culture serves as a frame of reference for one's perception and judgment and governs attitudes, reactions, health beliefs, and practices. People from one culture often differ from those in another culture in the way they think, solve problems or perceive the structure of the world.

Cultural orientation and background may be the most important factors to assess to understand the roles and functions within a family. Not all family members have the same emotional ties to their ethnic background. Older adults and parents who are in the process of raising children may adhere more closely to traditional values than adults without children.

If the cultural variable is not included as part of nursing assessment, misunderstanding may occur. Knowledge of a client's cultural heritage can provide insight and direction that lead to better client care and management. If the nurse is aware of the meaning of culture, a more holistic approach to care can be planned. Instead of making a snap judgment about a client's behavior the nurse will ask whether there is something about the client's cultural background that is affecting responses to health care.

ADULT

Recently, there has been an emphasis in the United States on searching for one's roots. This allows the adult to define his or her uniqueness in a "melting pot" of ethnic and cultural groups. Once role and cultural heritage have been defined, the adult educates his or her children regarding what the child must know or believe to behave in a manner that is acceptable to the family. Culture is not, therefore, an isolated concept; it is reflected in everything one says, does, and believes.

The manner in which beliefs, practices, habits, likes, dislikes, norms, customs, and rituals are transmitted and maintained within a particular family may be altered by political, economic, and social forces in our society. Nevertheless, essential components of the culture are usually passed along unaltered from one generation to the next.

OLDER ADULT

In many societies, the grandparents are vested with the responsibilities for passing on the cultural heritage to younger family members. Traditionally, the grandfather has been perceived as having the knowledge and patience to teach the younger men in the family cultural and ethical values learned over his lifetime that make his family unique. Grandmothers frequently function as role models and offer special teaching to the younger female family members so that traditions, beliefs and rituals are not lost from generation to generation. These teaching and sharing roles may provide a position of importance to the elders within the family or extended family and need to be assessed as part of the overall picture of family functions.

Differences in older people that have in the past been thought to be cultural in origin may have more to do with differences in educational level, socioeconomic status and language. Whatever the true source of these differences in older people, the nurse must always assess each client as an individual and plan nursing care accordingly.

EXPECTANT PARENT

In some cultures, reproduction is the way to achieve social status. During pregnancy, women are viewed as more attractive, receive more attention, and bring honor to the family. During the pregnancy there may be cultural restrictions placed on the mother. Certain indulgences must be avoided. These may include certain spices, foods, or sex. The pregnant client learns from her mother. Many feelings, attitudes, and health practices have firm cultural roots that affect the woman and the fetus. Often, health-care providers are not aware of the relationship of cultural patterns to the childbearing process. When people of different cultures enter the health-care-delivery system, cultural beliefs and practices are often overlooked. If their cultural values vary from the norm, these people may be viewed as different or strange. To facilitate holistic care, assessment of cultural needs and concerns during pregnancy and the birth process is very important. This is followed by attention during the postpartum period.

The roles of the members of the expectant family need to be assessed. In some cultures, women are responsible for the care of the woman in labor and even up to three months after delivery. Some cultures have defined rituals, taboos, and duties that must be performed by the father of the baby. For example, in some Native American cultures, the male is expected to make a cradleboard for the baby. These duties allow the father to establish his paternity and emphasize his responsibility to his family.

NEWBORN

The meaning or the value of the newborn within the culture will greatly influence the type of care given to the baby. Certain people may be assigned to care for bathing and dressing the baby. Certain family members or friends may choose the baby's name. Others may make a layette or purchase a crib. There are many rituals or ceremonies associated with the new baby. A boy may receive his name on the sixth day or be circumcised on the seventh day. In some cultures, babies may not be considered persons until after three months.

An important factor to consider in planning for the newborn is the question of circumcision and how it relates to the culture. The American Academy of Pediatrics (1975) stated that there is no medical reason to routinely circumcise the neonate. In many parts of the English-speaking world, however, this procedure is routine. Helping parents to decide about newborn circumcision from a cultural standpoint is a nursing responsibility. Discussion of circumcision should begin in the antepartum period. This allows the family to think about their rationale for deciding whether or not to circumcise their male newborn.

INFANT/CHILD/ADOLESCENT

Children readily learn the language of their parents, what foods to eat, and what behaviors and roles they perform within their family. Within cultures there are certain ways for children to behave; "children may be seen and not heard" or the entire family may focus on the behavior of the children.

The meaning of this baby to the family in relation to its culture will affect how the baby's needs are met and how the child is fed, groomed, and disciplined. It is generally felt that the cultural values that a child learns affect its attitudes and behaviors for life. Culture guides children and adolescents toward the development of meaning for the decisions that they make as adults.

QUESTIONNAIRE

ADULT

What is your country of birth?

Where did your parents or ancestors come from? When?

What are the habits, customs, beliefs and values of your culture? (Consider sex, surgery, health care, illness, death.)

What is restricted by your culture? (Consider sex, surgery, health care, illness, death.)

What language do you use in thinking?

What are some of the special things you do? (Consider holidays, holy days, birthdays, raising children.)

Does your family use folk medicine or traditional healers?

Is there a community health worker in whom you have confidence?

What does it mean to you to be healthy, to stay healthy, or to be sick?

Do you have specific practices for treating sickness or death, and if so, what are they? (Consider teas, herbs, poultices, other remedies.)

How does your culture respond to alterations in body image, change, stress, pain?

What language do you speak at home, at work?

Is the language spoken in your home now different from when you were a child?

Modifications for the Older Adult

Has identification with ethnic or cultural group changed or evolved in your lifetime?

Has this caused any conflict?

What place do you consider home?

What is the elder's role in health and illness?

Who is responsible for raising children?

Have your traditional roles and habits changed with age, and if so, how?

Modifications for the Expectant Parent

What role do the mother, father, grandmother, and other children play during pregnancy and childbirth?

Do you have beliefs about things that will harm the unborn baby?

What behaviors are accepted by your culture during pregnancy and childbirth?

Are the woman and man allowed to actively participate in the pregnancy and childbirth?

What are your cultural practices for pregnancy, labor and delivery, and postpartum period?

Do you have any dietary restrictions and sanctions during pregnancy?

Are there taboos or things that must be done during pregnancy?

Do you have beliefs about special things to eat or drink to find out the baby's sex or beliefs about things to eat or drink to make the baby male or female?

Do you use folk medicine during pregnancy; if so, for what conditions?

Modifications for the Newborn

Are there ceremonies to celebrate the birth?

Is the male or female child more valued?

Can the parents define circumcision?

Is the father circumcised?

Who made the decision about circumcision (mother, father, jointly) and why?

How did you obtain information about circumcision? (Consider classes, doctor, clinic, nurse, family.)

If there is a fetal demise, stillbirth, or infant death, determine cultural practices.

Modifications for the Infant/Child/Adolescent

What do you expect your child to do to assist with the needs of the family?

What are your jobs within the family?

Do you like the new baby?

Do you baby-sit and how often?

What are the kinds of things you eat every day? (Consider likes, dislikes, what the parent does, does not allow.)

What do you do to stay healthy and what do you do when you are sick?

REFERENCE

American Academy of Pediatrics Committee on Fetus and Newborn. Report of the ad hoc task force on circumcision. *Pediatrics* 1975, *56*, 610–611.

BIBLIOGRAPHY

Aamodt, A. M. *Social–cultural assessment of a child–nurse encounter in a health and healing scene.* Tucson, Ariz.: College of Nursing, University of Arizona, n.d.

Bauwens, E. E. *The anthropology of health.* St. Louis: Mosby, 1978.

Branch, M. F., & Paxton, P. P. (Eds.). *Providing safe nursing care for ethnic people of color.* New York: Appleton-Century-Crofts, 1976.

Brink, P. J. (Ed.) *Transcultural nursing: A book of readings.* Englewood Cliffs, N.J.: Prentice-Hall, 1976.

Brink, P. Value of orientations as an assessment tool in cultural diversity. *Nursing Research,* 1984, *33,* 198–203.

Brownlee, A. T. *Community, culture, and care: A cross-cultural guide for health workers.* St. Louis: Mosby, 1978.

Clark, A. *Culture, childbearing, health professionals.* Philadelphia: Davis, 1978.

Ebersole, P., & Hess, P. *Toward healthy aging.* St. Louis: Mosby, 1981.

Goodenough, W. Cultural anthropology and linguistics. In P. Gavid (Ed.), *Georgetown University round table on language and linguistics.* Washington, D.C.: Georgetown University Press, 1957.

Higgins, P. G., & Wayland, J. R. Labor and delivery in North America: A comparison between the native American and white cultures. *Nursing Times,* Midwifery supplement, 1981, *77.*

Hogstel, M. O. *Nursing care of the older adult.* New York: Wiley, 1981.

Humenick, S. Mastery, the key to childbirth satisfaction. *Birth and the Family Journal,* 1981, *8*(2), 79–83.

Kay, M. A. *Anthropology of human birth.* Philadelphia: Davis, 1982.

Leininger, M. *Transcultural nursing: Concepts, theories, and practices.* New York: Wiley, 1978.

Lynch, L. R. (Ed.). *The cross-cultural approach to health behavior.* Madison, N.J.: Fairleigh Dickinson University Press, 1969.

MacGregor, F. C. Uncooperative patients: Some cultural interpretations. *American Journal of Nursing,* 1967, *67*(1), 88–91.

Maheady, D. C. Cultural assessment of children. *American Journal of Maternal-child Nursing,* 1986, *11*(2), 128.

Moore, L. G. *The biocultural basis of health: Expanding views of medical anthropology.* St. Louis: Mosby, 1980.

Munroe, L., & Munroe, R. H. *Cross-cultural human development*. Monterey, Calif.: Brooks/Cole, 1975.

Orque, M., Bloch, B., & Monrroy, L. S. *Ethnic nursing care: A multicultural approach*. St. Louis: Mosby, 1983.

Spector, R. E. *Cultural diversity in health and illness*, 2nd ed. Norwalk, Conn.: Appleton-Century-Crofts, 1985.

Steele, S. M., & Harmon, V. M. *Values clarification in nursing*, 2nd ed. Norwalk, Conn.: Appleton-Century-Crofts, 1983.

Thiederman, S. B. Ethnocentrism: A barrier to effective health care. *Nurse Practitioner*, 1986, *11*(8), 52, 54, 59.

Thompson, J., & Bowers, A. *Clinical manual of health assessment*. St. Louis: Mosby, 1980.

Werner, E. E. *Cross-cultural child development: A view from the planet earth*. Monterey, Calif.: Brooks/Cole, 1979.

Whaley, L., & Wong, D. *Nursing care of infants and children*. St. Louis: Mosby, 1983.

UNIT 3

Environmental Safety

INTRODUCTION

Safety and security are basic human needs and are closely associated with the various environments in which one lives, works, and carries out various activities. In recent years, there has been emphasis on safety in the workplace as a result of the activities of the Occupational Safety and Health Administration (OSHA) in regulating more and more substances and circumstances that have been found to have detrimental effects on workers. Health hazards such as asbestos, noise, and radiation increase the mortality and morbidity rates. Limits now exist for acceptable exposures to many of these substances and conditions. As new hazards are discovered and documented, new standards are defined to protect the individual and the environment. It must be recognized, however, that new standards usually lag behind the identification of hazards.

Additional emphasis on environmental quality has come about as a result of efforts to have cleaner air and water. Industries that pollute the environment are required to install filtering and cleaning systems for air and water leaving manufacturing and industrial plants. Cities have been required to upgrade the quality of water in public supply systems. The Environmental Protection Agency of the federal government sets standards for the environment and imposes fines on violators.

Much research and effort have gone into decreasing the hazards of fire in our environment. Children's sleepwear is treated with substances that retard the rate at which it will burn. Attention has been given to the toxicity of fumes that are created by the burning of home furnishings and car and airplane interiors.

Causes of accidents are publicized by public service messages on radio, television, and other forms of communication in an effort to increase awareness of hazards to the health and general welfare of people. Accidents are the number-one killer of children and young adults, and most accidents occur in the home. For this reason, the nurse should assess the safety features of the home environment as well as community and work-related hazards.

Recently, there has been discussion of the environmental quality created in offices and restaurants as a result of the presence of persons who smoke. Nonsmokers must, of course, breathe smoke-filled air as well and are becoming quite vocal about their feelings in this matter. Smokers and nonsmokers have long been separated on airplanes. More and more restaurants have separate areas for nonsmokers. The battle lines are drawn between smokers and nonsmokers in offices where both are employed. Some employers hire only nonsmokers, whereas others have attempted to separate smokers from nonsmokers in the office. There is increasing concern about lung disease in children, spouses, and other family members where there is continuous smoking in the home.

The automobile has received a great deal of the attention of safety-minded persons for many years. As a result of this attention, the automobile as well as highways, streets and bridges are safer. We have shatterproof glass and seat belts and are now discussing the pros and cons of air bags in our cars. Many states have mandatory child-restraint laws; several states are also considering or have passed legislation that requires adults to wear seat belts. Better highway designs and surfaces have also been a part of the effort to decrease the rate of auto accidents.

The concept of a safe environment is a broad one that has many dimensions. Assessment of environmental safety requires the nurse to consider the various activities of each person and evaluate this in light of the individual's environmental well-being.

ADULT

The adult is responsible for his or her own environment and safety. It would seem to be a fairly easy task for the adult to provide for safety needs; however, there are many potential hazards beyond the control of one individual. Fear for safety does not usually concern the adult unless a severe stress has been experienced. Most adults feel they are at a peak both physically and emotionally, which can lead to a false sense of security and cause safety precautions to be taken for granted.

The automobile is one major area where the adult can modify accident potential that may result in death or severe injury. Three factors over which the client has control are seat-belt use, defensive driving techniques, and alcohol consumption while driving. The client who does not drink and drive and uses a seat belt while driving can dramatically reduce the risk of serious injury or death.

OLDER ADULT

For the older client, sensory changes as part of the aging process may slow the response and reaction time to various stimuli in the environment. This is particularly important when driving an automobile or operating other machinery. Vision and hearing changes as well as a slowed reaction time must be considered when evaluating whether the older person can continue to drive safely.

Falls are the leading cause of accidental injury in older persons, and generally there are many precautions that will help with prevention. Elimination of hazards in the home environment and adequate lighting are two important ways to decrease the incidence of falling. Clothing for elderly persons should be well fitted rather than loose or dangling. Shoes should not be soft or floppy. If the older person cannot bend down to tie shoelaces, slip-on shoes should be selected. Alterations need to be made in clothing as posture changes occur with aging, so that clothing does not drag or become hazardous in other ways. For example, if an elderly woman wears slacks, they should be shortened as she grows shorter because decreasing height is a part of the normal aging process.

The elderly are vulnerable and often victims of violence, both at home and in public places. The news frequently reports instances of purse-snatching from elderly women pedestrians, often in conjunction with personal injury. Life-styles of older persons should be assessed to eliminate as many of these potentially dangerous situations as possible.

EXPECTANT PARENT

The timing and mode of travel used by expectant parents should be discussed with the health-care provider as the later months of the pregnancy are reached. Generally, travel by car, train, bus, or air is without harmful effects, provided safety precautions are used. It is known that the use of seat belts reduces the number and severity of injuries resulting from automobile collisions for all persons including pregnant women. It should be remembered that in severe collisions, if the woman does not wear a seat belt, death of both mother and fetus frequently occurs by ejection from the car. If the mother wears a seat belt and a serious accident occurs, the potential is for the loss of one life rather than two.

NEWBORN

In today's highly mobile society the need to address the issue of auto safety is greater than ever. Automobile accidents are the leading cause of death in young children because approved child restraints frequently are not used in the car. The use of a restraint system properly anchored can reduce the incidence of fatal injury by a substantial amount.

Any safety restraint should have been approved by the National Highway Traffic Safety Administration, in accordance with the size or type of vehicle in which it will be used.

The selection of a car restraint is based on three factors—age, weight of child and whether or not the car seat requires a tether strap. The strap is the means by which the restraint may be properly installed in the automobile. If the cost of a car seat seems to be a deterrent for the family, the nurse can help the family contact local agencies or hospitals where low-cost car seats are available through rent or lowered purchase price.

INFANT/CHILD/ADOLESCENT

A safe environment is one of the greatest responsibilities a parent faces when raising a child. This requires careful planning and awareness of the abilities of the child. It is widely known that infants and toddlers have a high incidence of injury as a result of falls from which they could be protected. It is a good practice from the beginning never to leave the infant or small child unattended on any elevated surface. Crib railings should be up whenever the child is in the crib.

Many items are available that assist the care giver to "child-proof" the environment. These include plastic inserts for electric outlets, cabinet door and drawer latches, and toilet locks. Bath rings with suction cup legs are available to help prevent falls in the bathtub. High chairs and strollers are equipped with seat belts, which should always be used. However, even with a child-proof environment, the child must be carefully supervised. The nurse can encourage parents in this area.

Once the child is able to walk, he or she becomes very curious about the immediate environment and continues to explore it. Everything the child touches and feels usually goes into its mouth. Parents can help by selecting toys that are age appropriate and by not permitting a toddler to play with an older sibling's toys. The child further complicates matters by wanting everything it sees and so is constantly climbing to reach objects. Toddlers are fascinated by water and often play in it. The incidence of drownings in toilet bowls, buckets of water, and pools is high in this age-group. Toy manufacturers are aware of increased safety needs and have attempted to make toys of safer materials and designs as well as to indicate an appropriate age range for their use.

The preschooler is active and has not yet learned to think before acting. The young child learns by imitation, and this is a good time for the parent to begin safety teaching. Included in this teaching should be traffic, water and poison safety, as well as the safe use of toys.

During the school-age years children enjoy activities with other children. They are able to control impulsivity and begin to reason before they act. They like to be active, have less supervision, and may bicycle or participate in sports. A discussion of related safety precautions would include the necessity of appropriate clothing, safety gear and common sense when participating in these activities. The school-age child will also need instruction in traffic safety and recreational safety, which may include information on boating, swimming, or skating.

The child often comes into contact with strangers. This can be a potentially dangerous situation if the child does not understand the need to refuse offers of candy, requests to help a stranger, or offers of a car ride.

Adolescents have a high rate of accidents, the most common being automobile-related. Teenagers are risk-takers because their physical development is taking place rapidly, their life experiences are limited, and they have little sense of fear of new challenges or circumstances. The majority of time is spent away from the home. The teenager needs educational information on accident prevention. The educational goal for the teenager is that there be compliance with safety principles regardless of whether or not there is adult supervision. The teenager needs to take standardized driver education classes. If the instruction is provided by someone other than a parent, this may help to decrease the anxiety, anger and frustration that occasionally results when a parent does the teaching. A defensive driving course can be a good supplement to the standardized driver's education.

QUESTIONNAIRE

ADULT

Does your home have potentially dangerous structural or health problems? (Consider such things as plaster coming down from ceiling, stairway with boards missing, rodents.)

Are there hazards in your home? (Consider fire, stairs, inadequate heat, open gas heaters, inadequate toilet facilities, pest control, inadequate space, noise [television, radio], overcrowding [furniture, people].)

Are there hazards in your neighborhood? (Consider noise, water, and air pollution, police protection, heavy traffic on surrounding streets, isolation from neighbors, overcrowding.)

Are there community hazards? (Consider availability of stores, markets, laundry facilities, access to bus line.)

Are there safety hazards in your work environment? (Consider air and water pollution, noise, asbestos, radiation, chemicals, machinery, lighting.)

What measures do you take to reduce the risk of accidents and injuries in your home? (Consider smoke detectors, fire extinguishers, evacuation plan and alternate plan.)

Do you drink or use drugs while driving or operating machinery or ride with drivers who drink or use drugs while driving?

Do you wear seat belts and shoulder harnesses when driving and riding in the car?

Do you feel you drive safely?

Modifications for the Older Adult

Do you have assistance with household maintenance when necessary?

How do you carry valuables? (Consider women with handbags, man with wallet.)

Do you feel secure in your neighborhood?

Are there persons who are near and available if help is needed?

Does a trusted neighbor or friend have access to your house in case of emergency? (Consider key, garage-door opener, combination for lock.)

Do you have an established telephone network for safety and security purposes?

Is the environment arranged according to your abilities or disabilities? (Consider lighting, safety rails, throw rugs, clutter, wires, obstacles.)

Modifications for the Expectant Parent

Have you considered how your environment will affect your baby?

Does the seat belt or harness bother you when you ride in a car now that you are pregnant?

Do you feel that your sense of balance has changed now that you are pregnant and have you made any changes? (Consider shoes, style of dress.)

Modifications for the Newborn

What effect does the environment have on health status and developmental level of the newborn? (Consider lighting, noise, activity, color, variation.)

Does your infant travel in a car seat?

What type of car seat do you use for your infant?

Modifications for the Infant/Child/Adolescent

Is the child's environment safe and free of hazards? (Consider position of crib sides, area for crawling, rolling, exploring, clear floor areas, location of stairs, open windows, latches on screens and open doors, waxed floors, adequate supervision when on elevated surfaces [bed, counter top, changing table].)

Is the child's environment safe and free of burn hazards? (Consider vaporizer away from crib or bed, high chair out of reach of working and cooking surfaces, pans and tubs of hot water left unattended, pot handles out of reach.)

Is the environment child-proofed? (Consider location and storage of medicines, caustic and poisonous substances, accessibility of poisonous plants, appropriate covers for electrical sockets, location of fans and heaters, removal of tempting or sharp objects, overhanging table covers, accessibility of objects covered with lead-based paint, accessibility of pins, buttons and other small objects, checking toys for detachable small parts, use of gates at the top of stairs.)

Is the child's play environment safe and free of hazards? (Consider security fencing and supervision of the area and play activities.)

Does the child know what to do and say when approached by a stranger?

Does the child feel safe when left alone? (Consider working mother, no after-school supervision.)

BIBLIOGRAPHY

Andrews, A. W. Rural environment assessment: Implications for community health nurses. *Home Health Care Nurse,* 1985, *3*(5), 39–44.

Ebersole, P., & Hess, P. *Toward healthy aging.* St. Louis: Mosby, 1981.

Freudenberg, N. Citizen action for environmental health: Report on a survey of community organizations. *American Journal of Public Health,* 1984, *74*(5), 444-448.

Kozier, B., & Erb, G. L. *Fundamentals of nursing.* Menlo Park, Calif.: Addison-Wesley, 1983.

Pender, N. *Health promotion in nursing practice,* 2nd ed. Norwalk, Conn.: Appleton & Lange, 1987.

Pfeiffer, G. O., & Casimer, M. N. (Eds.). *The household environment and chronic illness: Guidelines for constructing and maintaining a less polluted residence.* Springfield, Ill.: Thomas, 1980.

Rivera, F. P. Epidemiology of childhood injuries. I. Review of current research and presentation of conceptual framework. *American Journal of Diseases of Children,* 1982, *136*(5), 399–405.

Schlapman, N. Concerns about passive smoking. *Journal of the American Association of Occupational Health Nursing,* 1986, *34*(4), 174–176.

Whaley, L. F., & Wong, D. L. *Nursing care of infants and children.* St. Louis: Mosby, 1983.

Wishon, P. M. Bicycles, roller skates and skateboards: Safety promotion and accident prevention. *Children Today,* 1986, *15*(3), 11–15.

UNIT 4

Exercise

INTRODUCTION

Regular exercise is an integral part of keeping healthy and fit. The fitness craze that is so prevalent at the present time has made it difficult for anyone to ignore the importance of exercise in making one feel and look good. But what are the actual benefits of exercise in terms of physical conditioning?

Effective exercise is aerobic and consists of ongoing physical activity that is repetitive and rhythmic, involving the use of large muscle groups. This type of exercise challenges the cardiovascular system by increasing the blood flow to the heart and thus increasing the heart rate. The strength of the cardiac muscle is improved, secondary to the increase in the heart rate. Aerobic exercise improves circulation throughout the body and increases the efficiency of the heart, lungs, and muscles.

Exercise helps the individual to relieve stress and tension and can also help one sleep better. Psychological well-being is improved through regular exercise as a means of stress reduction, and often the individual becomes optimistic and enthusiastic about life in general. Along with a proper diet, aerobic exercise helps to build endurance, firm muscles, and reduce or control weight because nutrients are more efficiently metabolized and utilized.

If aerobic exercise is to contribute to the fitness of the individual, it should be done for a minimum of 20 minutes three times each week. The exercise must also be strenuous enough to increase the heart rate to the target zone. The target zone is from 75 percent to 85 percent of the maximum attainable heart rate and is determined by the following formula:

$$(220 - \text{Age}) \times 75\% = \text{heart rate for 1 minute}$$

One repeats this formula using 85 percent instead of 75 percent, thus yielding the desired range for the pulse during exercise. (The formula is not suitable for persons who are taking heart-rate-altering drugs.)

Example for a 42-year-old target heart-rate range (Brody, 1982; Gasner & McCleary, 1982):

$$(200 - 42) \times 75\% = 134$$
$$(200 - 42) \times 85\% = 151$$

The target heart range, in this case 134 to 151, is the range in which exercise will be the most beneficial. If the pulse rate is above the target zone, the exercise should be considered too strenuous and the individual at risk for physical complications. No additional fitness is achieved by increasing the time spent exercising each day because the muscles begin to fatigue and utilize anerobic rather than aerobic metabolism after about 20 minutes of exercise. By increasing the frequency of the 20-minute period of exercise to four or five times per week, one can derive more benefits from the program.

Jogging, bicycling, walking, and swimming are examples of activities that are aerobic in nature. Isometric exercises and weight lifting may be used as an adjunct to the aerobic exercise program to improve muscle strength if necessary. It is important to remember that isometric exercises do not improve cardiovascular endurance, and they are not recommended for persons with cardiovascular diseases or problems.

Appropriate consideration of and planning for the possible problems an individual could encounter while exercising can prevent injury. The health and physical capabilities of the individual must be kept in mind so that the exercise program will not be harmful to health. To prevent aching feet and muscle strain the individual should have shoes that fit well and provide adequate arch support and cushioning for the structures of the feet. Clothing should be chosen with consideration for comfort of the individual, the environmental temperature, and the humidity.

Another important concept to keep in mind when designing an exercise program for the client is safety. A client who lives in a neighborhood with a high crime rate or one with no sidewalks or a lot of ice and snow may want to drive to a mall and take a brisk walk indoors rather than risk accident or injury.

ADULT

Careful selection of an exercise program that can easily be incorporated into the schedule of a busy adult is one of the major factors to keep in mind. The program should provide pleasure and enjoyment or in some other way be rewarding so that the individual will want to follow the program faithfully. This will help the individual toward development of a lifetime commitment to exercise. If the program is discontinued for a few weeks the beneficial effects are quickly lost. Exercising with a friend or family member is a good motivating factor for some people.

The goal of the adult's exercise program is personal fitness. Therefore, the exercise prescription for each person will be different. It will incorporate as many unique features of each individual's lifestyle, such as time the adult has to spend exercising each week, type of activity preferred, physical capabilities, availability and convenience of exercising equipment and facilities, and the environment in which the person lives.

The sedentary adult needs to have a complete physical examination, including electrocardiographic (ECG) stress testing, before beginning any strenuous exercise regimen. The adult who has had little or no exercise for many years needs to begin the program slowly to prevent injury. To begin a fitness program, for example, one could start by increasing the walking distance. The client could incorporate exercise into a busy schedule by parking the car one block away and then walking briskly to the office. Stairs can also be used instead of elevators. After becoming accustomed to this level of exercise the next step might be to begin light jogging or swimming for 10 minutes three times a week and work gradually up to 20-minute periods of more strenuous exercise. Many physicians recommend developing a walking pace that will achieve a 15-minute mile as an excellent exercise.

The weekend athlete is more prone to injury and illness related to exercise than the person who schedules exercise at regular intervals throughout the week. Continuation of the exercise regimen is required to maintain cardiovascular fitness.

OLDER ADULT

Among older persons there are those who have worked at manual labor for much of their lives and come to their retirement years with a satisfactory level of fitness. Others may have had various types of sedentary employment that contributed little to overall physical fitness. Exercise tolerance and personal stamina in this age-group may be altered in those with chronic disease or who have smoked cigarettes for many years. During working years, the person who is now retired may have been exposed to chemicals or other industrial hazards that have since been found harmful and placed under stricter control. A careful occupational history will yield many clues about these possibilities.

If the older person has had a regular exercise regimen for many years, most likely the same pattern will be carried over into retirement and perhaps enhanced or expanded as a result of having additional free time. If, however, it is necessary to begin the exercise program in the later years, this should probably be done under the supervision of a health professional because it must be carefully tailored to meet the needs of the individual. The plan must take into account interests and current health status. As one ages, exercises that involve coordination and flexibility need to be performed. Strength or endurance exercises should be encouraged. With aging, strength is lost in back and leg muscles more than arms, and this should be considered in planning the exercise regimen. There is, however, a general consensus that in the older person physiological functions and a sense of well-being are enhanced by regular exercise in much the same way as in younger populations.

EXPECTANT PARENT

Pregnancy should not interfere with the types of exercises a woman regularly enjoys. Even strenuous exercise done regularly by the woman before pregnancy can be continued provided it is not carried to the point of fatigue. If the woman is physically fit at the time she becomes pregnant, the respiratory and cardiovascular reserves are adequate to meet the needs of the fetus during the maternal exercise regimen if she stops exercising before becoming tired (Woodward, 1981). Exercises that involve body balance such as diving, surfing, and horseback riding should be avoided. Walking is still the best exercise and should be part of a daily regimen. Beginning a strenuous exercise program should be postponed until after delivery and planned with the health-care provider at the time of the postpartum checkup.

Exercise makes the pregnant woman feel good and helps prepare the body for labor and delivery. Muscular relaxation allows the woman to actively participate in the labor and delivery process. Practicing tightening and relaxation exercises during the pregnancy gives the woman some realization that she has control over her muscles and that she can learn to relax and use them fully for the birth of the infant.

NEWBORN

Exercise as we know it is not usually considered to be part of a new baby's life. However, stimulating exercises for the new baby are essential for both mind and body. The parent's face is a source of visual stimulation. The newborn is able to see most clearly when the parent's face is 7 to 8 inches from the baby's face. This eye-to-eye contact is extremely significant in parent–infant interaction.

Touch, as stimulation, is essential for normal growth and development. Neonates are not the same but are unique in their needs for various sources of stimulation. Parents need to begin to identify these needs so that they can develop plans for meeting them. Bright colors and different patterns and designs should be incorporated into the nursery. There should be musical toys, mobiles, and soft animals or dolls of different textures. Each aspect of the environment should offer some sort of stimulation to the newborn.

The neonate hears as well as an adult. High-pitched voices elicit increased motor activity and alertness and low-pitched sounds are soothing. The care giver can stimulate the infant's hearing, and the baby will respond to voice intonations. Talking to the infant also enhances the parent–infant interaction.

INFANT/CHILD/ADOLESCENT

During the early developmental years attitudes toward exercise are formed. If appropriate patterns of exercise are not formed during childhood and adolescence, the stage is set for a sedentary type of life-style in adulthood. It is the parent who influences the role exercise will play in the child's life. If exercise is an important part of the parent's life, the child will begin to value exercise as an integral part of his or her life-style.

As the young child develops, behavior is patterned after that of the parents. The child may say, "When I grow up I want to become a lawyer, just like Mommy and Daddy." Copying the behavior of their parents, younger children may dress up in their parents' clothes or play "house." It is easy to see that children learn by imitating the behavior of their parents. If a parent performs physical exercise daily, the child will be likely to emulate this behavior. Parents who walk, jog, or bicycle should encourage their children to participate along with them for both the fitness benefit and the benefit of spending time together as a family.

Unfortunately, health and physical education within the school system are not a national priority at the present time. Children spend one or two periods per week in performing exercises at school. Often these exercises are not aerobic. Emphasis is placed on noncontinuous group activities, team sports, and competition. In high school, physical education is often required only in the ninth grade, and after that the young person has the option of taking physical exercise as an elective course.

Issues of time and money affect how a school views health and exercise. One often hears "Lets get back to basics . . . kids need to have the three Rs." Health and physical exercise classes are one of the first to be cut in a school's budget. Health and physical education do not have to be expensive programs. Aerobic exercise programs that center around jogging, brisk walking, or running do not cost money and require only a little time and planning. Twenty minutes of well-planned physical activity each school day would meet the students' need for regular aerobic exercise. The value of exercise as part of a school's curriculum again relates to the aspect of parental attitudes and the value they place on exercise in the lives of their children. Parents, through their tax dollars and involvement in school activities, are able to influence what happens in school programs.

During the developmental years, there are appropriate exercises for each age level. It is not appropriate for a three-year-old to be in a jazz dance class, because of a lack of muscular development and rhythm coordination for such an advanced activity. Parents often feel that if their child is taking dancing lessons, doing gymnastics, or playing Little League baseball, the child is getting adequate exercise. These activities are important for the child to develop muscle tone and coordination and work in groups; however, they are not aerobic exercises.

If the adolescent is performing aerobic exercise, the young person should be praised for his or her behavior. This will foster and encourage the continuation of aerobic exercise. The school nurse and those who provide health and physical education activities need to become actively involved in setting up programs for those adolescents who are not involved in other aerobic exercise. Those things that are important to the adolescent need to be incorporated into programs. Emphasis on weight control, muscle tone, and firmness should be some goals for adolescent programs. The purpose of teen exercise programs should be to enhance the self-concept and body image.

QUESTIONNAIRE

ADULT

If age 35 or older, when was your last physical examination, including ECG stress testing?

Are there limitations on types of exercise you can do?

Do you know how to count pulse rate?

Do you know how to calculate your target zone?

What type of exercise do you do? (Consider type enjoyed, compatibility with life-style, warm-up, cool-down, intensity, duration, schedule, clothing, footwear.)

Do your daily activities include physical effort? (Consider moderate housecleaning, gardening, heavy lifting, moving heavy objects.)

Have you noticed any unpleasant effects with exercise? (Consider shortness of breath, fast heart rate for period of time greater than cool-down period, sore muscles and/or joints for extended periods of time.)

Modifications for the Older Adult

Are you able to take care of your home and yard?

Do you have any special health problems that influence your choice of exercise?

Who designed your exercise program?

Can you exercise now in the same way that you did in the past?

If exercise requires a partner (as in tennis) do you have difficulty locating someone?

Modifications for the Expectant Parent

Did you exercise regularly before pregnancy?

Has your exercise pattern changed since the pregnancy?

Has your exercise program been discussed with a health-care provider?

Were modifications or limitations suggested as pregnancy progresses?

How do you feel about exercise?

Do you and your partner attend prenatal (Lamaze) classes?

Modifications for the Newborn

How often do you allow the baby to move around freely? (Consider blankets, clothing, carrying devices, period of time and how often.)

How often do you exercise the newborn by playing with arms and legs?

How much time do you spend holding, touching, talking to your baby?

Modifications for the Infant/Child/Adolescent

Does your child pull himself to a standing position, practice crawling, walking?

How often do you hop, skip, dance, sing along with music?

Do you like your physical education classes? (Consider type of class and time spent.)

Tell me what you know about exercise?

Do your parents exercise regularly?

In what kind of competitive sports do you participate? (Consider how long, how often.)

REFERENCES

Brody, J. *Guide to personal health.* New York: Times Books, 1982.

Gasner, D., & McCleary, E. H. *The American Medical Association's book of heart care.* New York: Random House, 1982.

Woodward, S. L. How does strenuous maternal exercise affect the fetus? A review. *Birth and the Family Journal,* 1981, *8*(1), 17–24.

BIBLIOGRAPHY

Alexander, S. *Running healthy: A guide to cardiovascular fitness.* Brattleboro, Vt.: Stephen Greene, 1980.

American Heart Association. *'E" is for Exercise.* Dallas, Tex.: American Heart Association, 1977.

Burnside, I. M., Ebersole, P., & Monea, H. E. *Psychosocial caring throughout the life span.* New York: McGraw-Hill, 1979.

Delisa, J. A., & deLateur, B. J. Therapeutic exercise: Types and indications. *American Family Physician,* 1983, *28*(4), 227–233.

Department of Health Education. *Lifestyle assessment questionnaire.* Stevens Point, Wis.: University of Wisconsin, 1978.

Elmer-Deliutt, P. Extra years for extra effort . . . exercise can indeed increase longevity. *Time,* 1986, *127*(11), 66.
Finch, E., & Hayflick, L. *Handbook of the biology of aging.* New York: Van Nostrand Reinhold, 1977.
Hogstel, M. O. *Nursing care of the older adult.* New York: Wiley, 1981.
Jackson, C. P., & Brown, M. D. Analysis of current approaches and a practical guide to prescription of exercise. *Clinical Orthopaedics and Related Research,* 1983, *179,* 46–54.
Kopecki, R. A. Controlling stress in the home and the workplace. *Journal of the American Association of Occupational Health Nursing,* 1986, *34*(7), 314–322.
Larson, L. A., & Michelman, H. *International guide to fitness and health: A world survey of experiments in science and medicine applied to daily living.* New York: Crown, 1973.
Physical fitness and the older person: A guide to exercise for health care professionals. Rockville, Md.: Aspen, 1984.
Pollock, M. L., Wilmore, J. H., & Fox, S. M. *Exercise in health and disease: Evaluation and prescription for prevention and rehabilitation.* Philadelphia: Saunders, 1984.
Simkin, W. *The complete pregnancy exercise program.* New York: New American Library, 1980.
Timiras, P. S. *Developmental physiology and aging.* New York: Macmillan, 1972.
White, M. K. What the research says about exercise and osteoparosis. *Health Education Quarterly,* 1985, *16*(1), 3–5.

UNIT 5

Leisure Activities

INTRODUCTION

The life-style that an individual chooses can influence the quality and quantity of life. Throughout each day both mind and body are placed in stress-producing situations. Time must be allocated to restore the total self to harmony. Leisure activities that can be enjoyed alone or with others are one way to reduce stress levels. If this balance is not restored the individual, perceiving the stress to be harmful, may respond with behaviors that influence life-style. For example, with severe stress and no time for self, the individual may have difficulty remembering things because verbal information is not appropriately interpreted and assimilated. Without stress reduction one may also lose the ability to think clearly and have difficulty making decisions.

If there is no time allowance for participation in a leisure activity, stress will cause a disproportionate focus on self, and events may become magnified out of proportion. There is also a decrease in ability to cope with responsibility or to master tasks.

Periods of time should be allocated for recreation. Recreation is made up of various leisure activities that allow the mind and body to rest from the cares of family, business, or living. Everyone needs to put a little fun into life. If a person puts all available energy into work, home, and family and no time is allotted for leisure, the individual will eventually lose his or her effectiveness. When this condition is complicated by stress, the individual may feel worthless, incompetent, helpless, or lost.

ADULT

Adults may have many commitments and roles to perform and may lose sight of the importance of leisure time in restoring both body and mind. Leisure activities are one of the easiest things to eliminate from one's life to make time for career and family goals. These goals will be more easily attained when the adult recognizes the restoration of energy that can be derived from pleasurable activities.

OLDER ADULT

Theoretically, the older adult has more time for leisure activities because of retirement. In our society, however, retirement is poorly defined. Does it mean retirement from full-time work with pay to full-time volunteer work, or does one retire from full-time work to no work or only part-time work? Are we talking about retirement when one reaches age 65? What about the person who is still working at 72 years of age? It is important that the nurse not make assumptions about the average day of an older adult. Depending on the person's life-style, the older person may have just as much difficulty finding time for leisure activities as the younger one.

Because of our work-oriented society, some people reach retirement without having developed leisure activities that provide for enjoyment and stress reduction. More and more often, however, older people come to their retirement years having participated in various sports and hobbies and tend to continue these activities much as they did when they were younger. Some participate in a wider variety of leisure activities as they age. Membership of older adults in organizations probably decreases because of fewer dollars being available to cover these costs (Cutler, 1977).

In a 1976 study, Peppers found greater life satisfaction for older adults who were active after retirement than for those whose participation in activities decreased or remained unchanged as they aged. Life satisfaction, as one would expect, was greater for those who were doing what they most enjoyed. Changes or limitations in activities for the older client usually came about because of alterations in health status.

Like younger persons, the older adult may pursue hobbies in isolation or with others. Frequently, rewards come to the older person through opportunities to use old skills in new ways. Some develop leisure activities or hobbies to such an extent that they become financially profitable. Is it then work or leisure? Only a careful assessment will answer the question.

EXPECTANT PARENT

Leisure activities assume even greater significance during pregnancy. If this is a first pregnancy, often the woman has time on her hands, especially if she has left her job to await the birth of her baby. Women who have other children may feel trapped at home with the responsibilities of child care. In any case, time needs to be set aside for pleasurable pursuits. These may include family activities; however, the woman also needs time just for herself. Leisure, or free time, should be spent in whatever way the woman chooses to seek release from stress, responsibilities, or boredom.

The activities that the mother chooses should increase her self-esteem and feelings of worth as a person. During pregnancy the ego is often threatened. Changes in body image and psychological tasks of pregnancy affect the woman and her family. The woman needs to feel safe, secure, and have a sense of belonging. Recreation with friends and family helps to restore a sense of self and reestablish this sense of security and belonging.

NEWBORN

Pregnancy, childbirth, and childbearing are maturational crises. Each can produce stress for the new family. The new mother has a full-time job as care giver, wife, and mother. Without adequate help, she will suffer from lack of sleep and have little time to do family chores. With this added stress, the newborn can feel the mother's anxiety and react to the stress. The newborn may cry more or not settle down readily, thereby further increasing the mother's stress level.

New mothers need to be encouraged to schedule some time for themselves. They need to be encouraged to leave their infants in the hands of a caring person without feeling guilty. A planned trip to the store can be a tremendous lift to the psyche. Today many new mothers return to work soon after having their babies. Often there are feelings of anxiety and stress over leaving their babies. The nurse needs to reinforce the positive aspects of the quality of time the mother spends with the infant rather than the quantity of time. A component of this quality is the portion of time spent with the new baby as a part of the family unit. Both parents need to spend time with the baby aside from that time spent feeding, changing diapers, etc. This time over and above what is required to meet physical needs could be considered leisure time for the newborn. This time can be spent holding, watching, and talking to the baby. These activities allow the new family to get to know one another, learn about one another, and learn from one another in a safe, secure environment.

INFANT/CHILD/ADOLESCENT

From infancy through adolescence, play serves a variety of purposes and needs. For children, play may be directed or nondirected. That is, children may play alone or with others at their own pace. Children play to experience change, to explore the environment, to satisfy curiosity, and to experiment in a risk-free situation. The child may also be involved in directed play, such as participation on a soccer team. For the child who participates in this activity for enjoyment, it can be considered play as well as exercise. Play as a leisure activity may serve several purposes including selecting the activity, performance of or participation in the activity, and ultimately deriving pleasure from it (Craig, 1976).

When children start school, they have homework assignments and as they get older they should continue to be involved in outside-school activities. The adolescent becomes involved in still more activities, and school may become a full-time job. The child may need the help of his or her parents in finding time for leisure activities. Leisure/playtime activities enrich the life of each child by fostering intellectual development, interpersonal relationships, and problem-solving skills. Children also derive social skills and enhancement of creativity from playtime activities as well as developing social support groups. The sense of worth develops as a result of the interaction among childhood support groups and this can carry over into adulthood.

QUESTIONNAIRE

ADULT

Do you think leisure is important?

How much leisure time do you have?

Are you satisfied with the balance between work and play in your life?

Are you satisfied with the way you spend your leisure time?

What are your favorite leisure pastimes and/or other types of recreational activity? (Consider vocations, hobbies, sports [participator, spectator], music, language, travel [places, years], vacation, activity [what, for how long, how often], gardening, collecting.)

How often do you engage in recreational activity with family members?

Do you have any difficulty meeting the expenses involved in leisure or recreational activities?

Do you have other reasons for not participating in leisure activities?

Modifications for the Older Adult

Are you retired? (Consider adjustment, future plans, time spent in leisure/pleasurable activities.)

Do you feel safe going out during day, evening?

Is there someone to go with?

Do you have your own transportation; if not, what means do you use?

Do you belong to retiree or senior groups? (Consider political activity, veterans' organizations, volunteer work.)

Do you use a community or senior citizen center?

How do you relax and unwind?

Have your leisure activities changed?

Modifications for the Expectant Parent

How do you plan to spend your time before the baby comes?

How do you think the baby will change the daily activities of you and your partner?

When do you anticipate resuming former leisure activities?

Is there someone to help you when the baby comes home?

How long will they stay?

How will you divide up the chores?

How does the new father feel about changing diapers, feedings, less sleep, assuming some household duties?

What plans do you have for integrating leisure activities into your new schedule?

Modifications for the Newborn

Outside of physical needs, how much time do you and the father spend with the baby as a family?

How often do you leave the baby in the care of another and for how long?

How do you feel about leaving your baby with someone else?

Does your schedule set times to be away from your baby?

Do you plan to return to work?

Who will take care of your baby when you go back to work?

Modifications for Infant/Child/Adolescent

Does your infant play with hands, feet? (Consider rolling, changing positions, ability to amuse self, for how long.)

Do you feel it is important to hold and touch your child?

Does your infant have toy mobiles, noise-making objects, objects of various textures, bright colors, of visual interest and within reach?

How does your toddler use toys? (Consider car, telephone, tricycle.)

Does your toddler listen to short nursery rhymes and enjoy repetition? (Consider tactile stimulation, large picture books.)

Does your toddler initiate his or her own play activities, play alone better than with other children?

Do you play patty-cake, peekaboo with your toddler?

What kind of toys does your child play with during his or her bath?

Do you allow your child to play with other children?

Does your child imitate activities of parents?

Does your child actively play with toys and other materials without being encouraged?

What are your favorite toys, games, hobbies?

When you have a choice would you rather spend time doing things alone or with others?

REFERENCES

Craig, G. J. *Child development.* Englewood Cliffs, N.J.: Prentice-Hall, 1976, pp. 307–311.

Cutler, S. J. Agency and voluntary association participation. *Journal of Gerontology,* 1977, *32*(4), 470.

Peppers, L. G. Patterns of leisure and adjustment to retirement. *The Gerontologist,* 1976, *16*(S), 441.

BIBLIOGRAPHY

Butler, R., & Lewis, M. I. *Aging and mental health.* St. Louis: Mosby, 1982.

Carp, E. M., & Carp, A. Structural stability of well-being factors across age and gender, and development of scales of well-being unbiased for age and gender. *Journal of Gerontology*, 1983, *38*(5), 572–581.

Department of Health Education. *Lifestyle assessment questionnaire*. Stevens Point, Wis.: University of Wisconsin, 1978.

Godin, G. Assessment of leisure time exercise behavior by self-report: A concurrent validity study. *Canadian Journal of Public Health*, 1986, *77*(5), 359–362.

Hogstel, M. O. *Nursing care of the older adult*. New York: Wiley, 1981.

Mutran, E., & Reitzes, D. C. Retirement, identity and well-being: Realignment of role relationships. *Journal of Gerontology*, 1981, *36*(6), 733–740.

Noland, M. P. An empirical investigation of leisure exercise behavior in adult women. *Health Education*, 1985, *16*(5), 29–34.

UNIT 6
Nutrition

INTRODUCTION

Personal eating habits are determined by an interrelationship of factors such as culture, religion, social and economic status, individual preference, emotions, and health status. A nutritional assessment made by the nurse includes an evaluation of the physical and psychosocial components that affect nutrition. A balanced food intake is important to the total nutrition of the client and must take into consideration individual likes and dislikes. To maintain body weight and energy levels, the intake of nutrients should approximate the expenditure of energy. If there is an increase in intake and an individual has a sedentary life-style, obesity is a potential problem. On the other hand, with the emphasis in our society on the importance of being thin, many individuals have gone to the other extreme in inadequate nutrition and/or inappropriate weight reduction methods. Nutrition, exercise, and life-style need to be coordinated to maintain a stable body weight.

ADULT

A diet that provides calories in proportions of about one-half carbohydrates, one-third fats, and the remainder in protein is suggested for the normal adult. Daily calorie requirements vary depending upon life-style, with an active person requiring more calories than a sedentary one. A goal in the individual's life should be the maintenance of health and an appropriate body weight through a nutritious diet. To achieve this goal the individual will need to recognize and control any psychosocial factors that influence the intake of nutrients. For example, a hectic schedule for the person in the business world or a calendar with many social obligations may make eating a balanced diet difficult. Luncheon meetings, cocktail parties, and dinner engagements may increase the calorie intake without leaving enough time for a corresponding increase in exercise.

As the adult reaches middle age the basal metabolic rate decreases. To maintain body weight the adult must consume fewer calories or increase the amount of exercise to burn the calories. One of these activities or some combination of both will assist the adult in the goal of maintaining an appropriate body weight.

OLDER ADULT

The literature on nutrition for the older adult points out that nutritional factors influence the aging process as well as illness and that secondary diseases in the elderly can be prevented or influenced by diet (Roe, 1983). Sensory changes in the elderly that affect nutrition include impaired taste, particularly for salt and sugar. In the attempt to make food taste more palatable, salt or sugar is added to foods, which may exaggerate health problems. Chewing of food has a close relationship to nutrition for the older person; mastication may be impaired, as it is related to several chronic diseases, some of which are common in elderly persons. Periodontal disease may also be a factor in mastication because of the related inflammation of the gums and loosening of the teeth.

Older people often have problems with gut mobility, which has a relationship to nutritional status. The older person may become concerned with constipation and take a laxative, which begins a cycle of disruption of absorption of nutrients from the intestinal tract. Malnutrition of dietary or disease origin is not an uncommon occurrence in elderly people.

The older person, up to age 75, is generally thought to need approximately 90 percent of the adult requirement of essential nutrients. For those older than age 75, the present requirement is about 75 to 80 percent of the adult requirement, with 12 percent of the calories provided by protein. Large doses of vitamins are not recommended because they may pose health risks, including toxicity caused by the wide variations in rates at which the drugs are metabolized. A broad selection of foods from the different food groups will provide ensurance against a dietary deficiency of essential nutrients (Roe, 1983).

The present recommended dietary intake for the older person includes:

Food Group	Number of Servings
Dairy products	2
Meat and protein-rich	1 to 2
Vegetables and fruits (including juices)	4
Cereal and grains	4

Requirements for adequate nutrition in the elderly person are also dependent on drug intake and, to some degree, exposure to sunlight. Because exposure to sunlight is required for synthesis of vitamin D, these vitamins may need to be supplemented if the person has little sun exposure.

Though much of what has been discussed here has to do with physiological function in the elderly person, it is closely associated with the psychosocial aspect of nutritional status in the elderly person and must be kept in mind as the assessment is made. The elderly, as well as other groups in our society, have food preferences that are associated with cultural factors such as ethnicity, traditional or religious beliefs, and traditions within the family. Elderly persons are usually more rigid in their food preferences, and this can present real challenges to the nurse who must attempt to alter their diet.

Financial resources may also dictate food choices to some extent. If the elderly person must depend on social security alone for financial support in retirement, careful questioning about eating habits, diet, and shopping for food is appropriate. One may find that as the month passes the quality of nutrient intake is decreased. There may be no additional funds for food until the next social security check arrives.

Factors such as mobility must be considered in the nutritional assessment of the older adult. Can the person walk well enough to push the grocery cart through the store and stand long enough to complete the shopping? Does the older person have the necessary equipment for food storage and preparation? Is vision good enough to see the labels on the food as well as the controls on the range and refrigerator at home? The distance to the store must be evaluated as well as the transportation and the means to carry the groceries home. If it is a small neighborhood grocery, is there a variety of food available and are prices in line with larger supermarkets? If there is disability or a disease process present, there may be additional constraints relating to purchasing, preparing, and consuming appropriate essential nutrients.

Does the older person live alone so that socialization processes that we relate to mealtimes are absent? If so, is the problem compounded by lack of availability of small packages of food so that the same food must be eaten again and again or else discarded?

Several efforts have been made by governmental agencies to meet real or perceived nutritional needs in the elderly. Examples of these are congregate nutrition sites and Meals-on-Wheels programs. Usually these provide one meal a day, five days a week, and some have provisions for one meal a day over the weekend.

EXPECTANT PARENT

Prenatal nutrition is important because research shows that inadequate diets during pregnancy are associated with a higher incidence of complications during the pregnancy and delivery, as well as increased threat to the fetus and to long-range development of the child. Women who are well nourished decrease the incidence of stillbirths, prematurity, and congenital defects. A careful diet history of the pregnant woman will reveal whether the diet includes the recommended number of servings from the basic food groups for pregnancy and lactation.

The daily energy requirements of the woman during the first part of pregnancy are within the range for a nonpregnant client, about 2000 to 2100 calories a day. An increase to 2300 calories should occur during the third trimester, with an increase to 2500 calories if the mother is breast-feeding. It is impossible to recommend average weight gain for all expectant mothers. Some mothers are underweight; others are overweight. Generally, in an uncomplicated pregnancy, weight gain is about 3 to 4 pounds during the first trimester, 12 to 14 pounds in the second trimester, and 8 to 10 pounds during the third trimester. The daily allowance for protein during pregnancy is 76 grams. This is a 30-gram increase from the nonpregnant requirement. For lactation, 66 grams is required. If the mother is at high risk, an increase to 100 grams is appropriate. The mother should also be taking a multivitamin preparation. There is need to increase calcium (1.2 g/day), phosphorus (1.2 g/day), and iron (18 g/day) (Bobak & Jensen, 1987).

NEWBORN

Infants usually establish their own feeding schedule, often referred to as demand feeding. The new baby may require 10 to 12 feedings every 24 hours. Then an interval pattern develops, from 3 to 4 hours between feedings. During feedings, the care giver should be in a comfortable position and hold the baby close enough for the baby to feel comforted and to allow ease in swallowing. Feeding time is a special time for the care giver to learn about the baby and how he or she responds. The baby learns about the parent or care giver through the various senses and through this interaction builds a positive relationship.

Parents' choice between breast- or bottle-feeding for the newborn is no longer dictated by cultural norm or economic necessity in our society. There is, however, a growing movement back to breast-feeding for the first several months of the baby's life. If the woman plans to return to work, she may continue breast-feeding by using a breast pump to express milk during the time she is at work. This requires a little time, privacy, and a place to store the milk. Breast milk can be frozen for future use (Lawrence, 1985). Breast milk should be thawed in a pan of warm water at room temperature; it should not be placed in a microwave because high-intensity heat destroys the protein molecules in breast milk.

INFANT/CHILD/ADOLESCENT

Infants are usually introduced to foods on a gradual basis, with mothers giving a specific food at a specific age. Foods for the infant should, however, be introduced when the baby is ready to eat, not on the basis of some previously developed criterion or schedule. The bland foods, such as cereals with iron, should be introduced first, followed later by foods with fiber and complex proteins. Foods can be introduced one at a time in small amounts (1/4 teaspoon) and offered when the infant is hungry before the formula. Each new food should be offered several times in succession, rather than changing the items regularly, so that if there is a problem with digestion or allergy the cause can be easily discerned. By one year of age, the infant should have tasted some solid foods.

The toddler will enjoy eating finger foods, and the parent should not be concerned about messy eating efforts. The child who is able to manipulate smaller objects is ready to begin learning to use a spoon. It will take practice and time for the child to do a good job of feeding him- or herself. The toddler will be most successful when eating if there is a regular routine, with the child placed in a high chair and given small servings of food. If the child refuses to eat any particular food, that food should be removed and no attempts made to force the child to eat. The child may also eat only small amounts of foods at one sitting, and once the child demonstrates lack of interest in the food, no additional effort should be made to give more. The child in this age-group learns very quickly how to manipulate adults with the rejection of foods.

It is during the school-age years that peer groups and advertisements begin to influence the child's eating patterns, and eating junk foods may begin. The school-age child may become busy with social activities, such as sports or music after school, and eating may take the form of snacking. In this case, it is important to encourage nutritious foods for the snacks.

A tremendous growth spurt and physiological changes take place during the adolescent years so that the teenager requires an increase in nutrients to meet the metabolic requirements. Appropriate ranges of nutrients for the adolescent include protein (44 to 54 g), calories (2100 to 3000), calcium (1200 mg), and iron (18 mg) (Whaley & Wong, 1983). The peer pressure that began earlier in the school years has an even more profound influence on the eating patterns of the adolescent. The need to be the same as the rest of the group can lead to poor nutrition during this time of fast growth.

The adolescent girl may not be encouraged to participate in physical activities as much as her male counterpart. This, along with the deposition of fat in the female adolescent, predisposes her to obesity.

As a result, adolescent girls frequently go on crash diets to lose weight quickly. Therefore, it is appropriate for the nurse to assess the adolescent girl regarding her eating habits in relation to her feelings about herself as well as any possible overeating or anorexia.

QUESTIONNAIRE

ADULT

How would you describe your appetite? (Consider excellent, good, fair.)

Are your mealtimes regular every day?

How often do you eat three meals a day?

Where do you usually eat?

With whom do you usually eat?

What kind of snacks do you eat?

Do you eat breakfast? If not, when do you first eat and what do you eat?

What time of day do you eat your main meal on weekdays and weekends?

What special ethnic foods do you eat?

Do you have any current or past problems related to nutrition?

What vitamin or mineral supplements do you take?

Are there any particular foods you do or do not eat, and why? (Consider allergy, religion, cost, availability.)

Do you eat anything that is not considered food? (Consider clay, dirt, starch.)

Are there any foods you eat when you are sick?

Are you on any special diet? (Consider kind, by whom prescribed, for what purpose.)

Have you had any recent appetite changes? (Consider perception of reason, resulting weight change.)

Do you have adequate cooking equipment? (Consider range, microwave, small appliances, pots, pans.)

Do you have any difficulty in preparing food? (Consider physical disability, mental health, inadequate equipment, inability to prepare special diets.)

Who does the meal planning and cooking?

Do you add salt when preparing foods?

Do you usually use frozen, canned or fresh foods?

List the amounts and types of food or beverage you eat and drink from the time you get up in the morning until you go to bed and what you eat during the night. Keep this diary for 3 days.

What is your present weight; average over last year; average weight over the last 5 years?

Were weight changes rapid or slow?

How much weight lost or gained and over what period of time?

Have you ever been very over- or underweight? When and how much?

Do you have any difficulty chewing food? (Consider dentures [fit], oral pathology, condition of teeth, gums, buccal mucosa, when last seen by a dentist.)

Where is food obtained? (Consider homegrown [eaten fresh, canned, frozen]; if purchased, kind of store, budget/funds, distance, transportation, who shops, how often.)

How much do you spend on food each week?

How many people does this feed?

Do you have adequate food storage space? (Consider cabinets, refrigerator, freezer.)

Modifications for the Older Adult

Does your food taste as good as usual?

Do certain foods taste bad and if so, what foods?

Have you added any seasonings to make food taste better and if so, what and how much?

Are there foods you're not able to chew? If yes, which ones?

Are there foods that you are not able to swallow? If yes, which ones?

Do you have enough money for food?

Do you get Meals-on-Wheels? If so, how often?

How do you like the meals?

Do you eat at senior citizens' meal sites? If so, how often?

Can you see well enough to cook safely and operate the range?

Are you able to walk and stand long enough to prepare food?

Does your 3-day food diary represent changes from the recent past?

Modifications for the Expectant Parent

Have you craved any special foods? If so, what?

How much weight do you think you should gain with this baby?

Is this your first pregnancy? If not, how many others have there been?

When was your last baby born?

Does anyone in your family or the father's family have twins?

Have you had any nausea and/or vomiting with pregnancy?

How often do you take calcium supplements, vitamins, minerals?

Does your diet include iron-rich foods and supplements? (Consider raisins, liver, leafy green vegetables.)

Did you have any special diet during any previous pregnancy?

Now that you are pregnant, are there any foods you cannot eat?

Have you had elevated blood pressure or anemia with other pregnancy?

What was your weight before pregnancy?

What is your height and present weight?

What are your plans for feeding your infant? (Consider formula, breast-feed, undecided.)

Have you bottle- or breast-fed your other children and were there any problems?

What role will the father play in feeding the baby?

How often do you think your baby will eat?

Modifications for the Newborn

Is the baby breast- or bottle-fed?

Do you hold the baby during feeding?

How do you feel about feeding the infant in bed with the bottle propped?

Is your baby interested in eating?

Who feeds the baby?

What does the baby do after eating?

How does your baby suck?

How long does it take your baby to finish a bottle?

Does your baby suck his thumb or a pacifier?

Do you use your breast as a pacifier if the baby is upset or ill?

Do you have any concerns about your baby's nutrition or feeding habits?

How many ounces does your baby drink in a 24-hour period?

How often do you feed your baby?

Have you introduced solid foods? (Consider what, when, how much currently consuming per 24 hours.)

Modifications for the Infant/Child/Adolescent

Does your child eat alone or with the family?

Who feeds the child?

When is the child most hungry?

How long does it take your child to eat a meal?

Are your child's eating habits similar to those of other family members?

How does your child accept new foods?

How do you feel about using food as a punishment or reward?

How does your child behave at mealtime?

Do you have "clean plate" or "taste everything" rules?

Does your child care for own needs at the table? (Consider serving own food, finish all food, ask for second helpings, know when full, get up during the night to eat or drink.)

How do you feel about your body, too thin, too fat?

Do you follow any special diet? (Consider adherence, eating candy, desserts, or gum chewing.)

What fast foods do you eat and how often?

What is your favorite fast food restaurant?

Where do you have lunch on school days?

REFERENCES

Bobak, I., & Jensen, M. *Essentials of Maternity Nursing: The Nurse and the Childbearing Family* (2nd ed.). St. Louis: Mosby, 1987, pp. 593–595, 602, 621.

Lawrence, R. A. *Breastfeeding: A guide for the medical profession* (2nd ed.).St. Louis: Mosby, 1985, pp. 459–460.

Roe, D. A. *Geriatric nutrition.* Englewood Cliffs, N.J.: Prentice-Hall, 1983, pp. 18–24.

Whaley, L., & Wong, W. *Nursing care of infants and children.* St. Louis: Mosby, 1983, p. 691.

BIBLIOGRAPHY

Christakes, G. Nutritional assessment in health programs. *American Journal of Public Health,* 1973, *63,* 1–82.

Dawson, J. Nutritional assessment. *Journal of Gerontological Nursing,* 1986, *12*(3), 37.

Drugay, M. Nutritional evaluation: Who needs it? *Journal of Gerontological Nursing,* 1986, *12*(4), 14–18.

Fox, J. A. *Primary health care of the young.* New York: McGraw-Hill, 1981.

Goodinson, S. M. Assessment of nutritional status. *Nursing* (London), 1986, *3*(7), 252–258.

Hertzler, A. A., Wenkam, N., & Standal, B. Classifying cultural foods habits and meanings. *Journal of the American Dietetic Association,* 1982, *80*(5), 421–425.

Howard, R., & Herbold, N. *Nutrition in clinical care.* New York: McGraw-Hill, 1982.

Keithley, J. Proper nutritional assessment can prevent hospital malnutrition. *Nursing 79,* 1979, *9*(2), 68–72.

Kozier, B., & Erb, G. *Fundamentals of nursing concepts and procedures.* Menlo Park, Calif.: Addison-Wesley, 1983.

LeClerc, H. L., & Thornbury, M. E. Dietary intakes of Title III meal program recipients and nonrecipients. *Journal of the American Dietetic Association,* 1983, *83*(5), 573–577.

Malasanos, L., Barkauskas, V., & Stolenberg-Allen, K. *Health assessment.* St. Louis: Mosby, 1981.

Patten, S. E. Nutrition and the elderly: A cultural perspective. *Geriatrics,* 1982, *37*(5), 141–144.

Pearson, A. Nutrition in the middle years of childhood. *American Journal of Maternal Child Nursing,* 1977, 2(6), 383.

Riordon, J. *A practical guide to breastfeeding.* St. Louis: Mosby, 1983.

Roberts, B., Vermeersch, J., & Williams, S. *Nutrition in pregnancy and lactation.* St. Louis: Mosby, 1981.

Schwerin, H. S., Stanton, J. L., Smith, J. L., et al. Food, eating habits, and health: A further examination of the relationship between food eating patterns and nutritional health. *American Journal of Clinical Nutrition,* 1982, *35*(5 Suppl), 1319–1325.

Sorenson, K., & Luckman, J. *Basic nursing: A psychophysiologic approach.* Philadelphia: Saunders, 1979.

Stronmeyer, S. L., Massey, L. K., & Davison, M. A. A rapid dietary screening device for clinics. *Journal of the American Dietetic Association,* 1984, *84*(4), 428–432.

UNIT 7

Sleep

INTRODUCTION

Biorhythms or metabolic clocks are part of our makeup. The biological clock is controlled within the body and is altered slowly as environmental factors change. The wake-sleep cycle is an example of a human biological rhythm. Examples of situations that force changes in these rhythms include the change to daylight saving time, travel to other time zones, particularly across the international date line, or a work shift change from days to nights. Biorhythms are also referred to as diurnal or circadian because the length of the cycle is one day. The cycle varies somewhat from individual to individual, as evidenced by differing amounts of sleep required by each person, as well as the fact that some people function better in the morning, whereas others do their best work in the evening hours.

Sleep is a basic requirement of every human being. We cannot function appropriately without it, as evidenced by our spending more than one-third of our lifetime in this state. We know little about the mechanisms and function of sleep, but it is thought to be both a physical and mental restorative process. During this period information is stored and categorized by the brain, stress and anxiety are decreased, and the energy to cope with the daily tasks of life is restored. Sleep was at one time defined as a state of unconsciousness, but it is now known to be a characteristic state of consciousness. The ability of the person to perceive and react to appropriate internal and external stimuli indicates that the individual is not unconscious during this period but rather in an altered state of consciousness.

Many factors influence both the quantity and quality of our sleep. Some of these include age, personality, environment, exercise, hormones, foods and beverages, medications, tension, fatigue, illness, and alterations in patterns of daily living. One or more of these factors may be at work in an individual at any given time.

ADULT

The amount of sleep required by the adult varies according to the energy expended. The requirement for sleep is, in part, determined by biophysical, emotional, sociocultural, and environmental circumstances. Adults usually are busy trying to keep up with jobs, families, and community and recreational activities and, as a result, usually sleep 7 to 9 hours each night. However, the stresses imposed by the life-style that are inadequately controlled may lead to insomnia and thus to fatigue. This can be overcome by developing a good sleep preparation routine, relaxing at bedtime, creating an environment that is conducive to sleep, and getting an adequate amount of physical exercise.

OLDER ADULT

For the older person, sleep provides necessary restorative and recuperative functions. The older adult requires more rest during any 24-hour period but less sleep. Usually 5 to 7 hours of sleep are considered adequate for the well elderly person. Frequently, these people sleep less soundly and may have sleep interrupted by such things as nocturia, noise, tremors, unpleasant dreams, or muscle cramps in the legs. Many aged people have difficulty falling asleep, and patterns of insomnia should be carefully assessed. Inability to fall asleep at bedtime may indicate anxiety, whereas early awakening with inability to go back to sleep is often related to depression. Drastic alterations in sleep patterns may indicate serious illness.

All too often sedatives and hypnotics are prescribed for older persons who report sleep interruption. The older person is more susceptible to barbiturates because of further depression of bodily functions, lowering of the basal metabolic rate, and decreasing mental activity that may be already slowed as part of the aging process. Because of the longer half-life of drugs in the older individual, the effects of sedatives may carry over into the daytime hours and present as sluggishness and confusion. Rapid eye movement sleep (REM) is the most active period of sleep and the time during which dreams occur. Sedatives and hypnotics frequently alter or stop REM sleep, which decreases the quality of sleep and its related functions at a time in life when the quality of sleep also has an age-related decline.

The amount of stage four, or deep, sleep is decreased or absent in older persons. Long periods of wakefulness at night are not uncommon. Some of this sleeplessness may be related to medications being taken by the older person (i.e., diuretics, tranquilizers) or caused by dozing for extended periods throughout the day. Napping, as differentiated from dozing, is a deliberative process that occurs during the day. The nap is usually from 15 to 60 minutes long and, though it provides rest and relaxation, will usually interfere with night sleep to some extent. Other factors that may disrupt sleep in older persons are changes in sounds, mattress, or temperature. Bedtime rituals that facilitate sleep in older persons should be encouraged to help them have enough rest and sleep.

EXPECTANT PARENT

From the beginning of pregnancy there is an alteration in metabolic requirements, thereby increasing the need for sleep. During pregnancy, sleep helps facilitate adaptive responses. The pregnant client needs approximately 8 hours of sleep, with rest periods in the afternoon. The expectant mother should recognize the potential for increased fatigue and not stand when she can sit or sit when she can lie.

Toward the end of pregnancy, the enlarged uterus makes sleeping difficult. Extra comfort measures may be necessary to facilitate sleep. These might include any methods previously used effectively against insomnia plus a side-lying position with pillows to comfortably cushion abdomen and legs.

After the mother takes her new baby home her usual sleep patterns are disrupted. She will have changes and adjustments in her schedule as she cares for the newborn and often other responsibilities to family members. She should be encouraged to rest when she can and allow some time for herself so that she can have the opportunity to feel renewed and meet some of her own needs.

NEWBORN

Newborns can be expected to sleep from 18 to 22 hours per day. The newborn may move mouth and limbs during sleep and will usually awaken about every 4 hours to eat and then go back to sleep. Each infant develops a recognizable sleep cycle. Many a new mother's self-confidence and sense of adequacy is threatened when she feels she is unable to cope with her new baby and his or her sleeping patterns. Often the problem is that the mother may not understand the effect of her own anxiety on the infant. As the infant senses her tension, sleep may become more disrupted. By knowing that the infant responds in accordance with her emotional state, the mother can discipline herself to be more relaxed and at ease and thus have more enjoyment in caring for the new baby.

INFANT/CHILD/ADOLESCENT

During the toddler years the child requires about 10 to 14 hours of sleep a night and takes an afternoon nap. Toddlers may assert their independence by refusing to sleep or nap. Bedtime and naptime rituals become important during the toddler years. The child may need to have a story read aloud, say a prayer or brush his or her teeth before going to sleep. These rituals are highly individualized.

The school-age child sleeps from 9 to 13 hours each night. The most common sleep problems encountered during the school-age years are nightmares and sleepwalking. These are usually outgrown as the child gets older. The child who has nightmares needs to feel comfortable and secure because nightmares are a frightening experience. The child needs time to express feelings about the nightmare. Cuddling by the parent and a night-light in the child's room and hallway also serve to increase feelings of security while decreasing fears. Safety is the primary concern for the child who sleepwalks. The safety factors to be investigated are individualized depending upon the child's environment.

The adolescent usually requires from 8 to 10 hours of sleep each night. An additional rest or nap period may also be required because of the rapid growth and concomitant increase in energy expenditure during this time. The adolescent may need assistance to adjust a busy schedule so that he or she can get enough sleep, or the parents may need to be educated about the teen's sleep requirements so that they realize that the adolescent requires the sleep and is not lazy or shirking responsibilities.

QUESTIONNAIRE

ADULT

How many hours do you sleep each night, in each 24-hour period (exclude waking time spent in bed)?

Is this too much, too little, about right?

In your view do you sleep well?

Do you have any problems with sleep? (Consider getting to sleep, time to fall asleep, waking up, getting up in the morning, feeling fresh upon awakening, sleepiness during the daytime.)

How much does your bedtime vary? (Consider weekdays, weekends, holidays.)

When falling asleep do you have any problems? (Consider racing thoughts, feelings of sadness or depression, anxiety, muscular tension, muscle jerks, fear, pain.)

When going to bed, do you use any sleep rituals? (Consider earplugs, eyeshades, music, other sound, night-light, or any other bedtime rituals.)

Do you use any sleep aids? (Consider sleeping or other medication [complete that portion of medication assessment], hypnosis, baths, massage, sex, exercise, smoking, alcohol consumption.)

How often do you sleep with someone else? (Consider in room, in bed.)

Do you sleep on a special surface? (Consider bed board, mattress, water bed.)

How often do you have disturbed sleep? (Consider providing assistance to a child, ill person or pet; room temperature, light, noise, bed partner.)

How many times do you awake during a typical night? (Consider the longest period of time awake, which third of the night [first, middle, last], number of times out of bed during a typical night, why—hunger, thirst, voiding [number of times].)

Do you walk, talk during sleep, grind teeth, bang head on pillow or wall, make rocking, rolling movements, fall out of bed while asleep?

Do you snore? (Consider breath-holding, cessation of respiration during sleep.)

At what time of day do you function best?

Are there rest periods in your usual work day? (Consider length, frequency.)

Do you nap during workday? (Consider how many times, for how long, feel refreshed.)

What things affect your sleeping habits? (Consider food, beverage, exercise, stress, anxiety, fatigue, daytime rest or sleep, noise, weather, heat, cold, travel, work, physical problems, illness.)

Do your sleeping problems go in cycles? (Consider if sleep is abnormal, insomnia is present, problems better, worse in the past.)

How often do you have vivid dreams or nightmares? (Consider waking from a dream, having recurring, sleep-disturbing dreams, awake at same time.)

What time do you awaken on weekdays? (Consider time of arising, awake with alarm, difficulty awaking in the morning, sleeping past "getting-up time."

How long does it take to "get going" after arising? (Consider feeling of alertness, energy during the day, sleepiness during the day, falling asleep in spite of efforts to stay awake, fatigue present during the day, with or without sleepiness.)

Do you fall asleep without intending to? If so, during what activities?

Modifications for the Older Adult

Have you experienced sleep changes in recent years?

Do you nap more often than when you were younger?

Are there health problems that affect your sleep?

With change in work schedule, is there a better quality of sleep when working one schedule as opposed to another?

Modifications for the Expectant Parent

How has pregnancy changed your or your partner's sleep habits?

Can you rest during your pregnancy?

How much time are you up at night with other children? (Consider how long, frequency, difficulty getting back to sleep.)

Are you able to rest during the day as a compensatory measure?

Modifications for the Newborn

Where does your baby sleep?

How long does your baby sleep?

What kinds of things help your baby to get back to sleep?

Is your baby alert and active when awake?

Do you nap when your baby does?

Modifications for the Infant/Child/Adolescent

Does your child's sleep pattern interfere with family activities?

Does your child nap? How long, when?

Is the child fussy upon awakening or alert and active?

Does your child frequently spend the night away from home or have other children in for the night?

Does your child express fears of the dark or going to sleep?

Does your child sleep with the light on or with a favorite toy?

If parents are out for an evening does a familiar person who knows the sleep habits care for the child?

Does the child sleep in your bedroom or bed?

What do you do when your child awakens at night? (Consider taking into parents' room, discipline, comfort measures.)

BIBLIOGRAPHY

Brady, D. Health maintenance and promotion of the nervous system. In Bectell, P. *Health maintenance and promotion across the lifespan.* Norwalk, Conn.: Appleton & Lange (to be published).

Ebersole, P., & Hess, P. *Toward healthy aging.* St. Louis: Mosby, 1981.

Erman, M. K. Sound sleep; alcohol not an ingredient. *Journal of the American Association of Occupational Health Nursing,* 1986, *34*(6), 294–295.

Hoskisson, J. *What is this thing called sleep?* London: Davis-Plynter, 1976.

Mendelson, W. B. Sleep after forty. *American Family Physician,* 1984, *29*(1), 135–139.

Miles, L. *Sleep questionnaire and assessment of wakefulness.* Stanford, Calif.: Stanford University Medical Center, n.d.

Quan, S. F., Bamford, C. R., & Beutler, L. E. Sleep disturbances in the elderly. *Geriatrics,* 1984, *39*(9), 42–47.

Sorensen, K., & Luckman, J. *Basic nursing: A psychophysiologic approach.* Philadelphia: Saunders, 1979.

UNIT 8

Emotional Health

INTRODUCTION

An examination of the client's mental status occurs as a basic part of the complete physical assessment. Beyond that, however, there are psychosocial factors relating to emotional health that one must also assess in evaluating the function of any individual from a holistic viewpoint. Emotional health is a state of mind, relative to age and developmental tasks, that allows the individual to cope with the ongoing stresses of everyday life in a manner acceptable to him- or herself and significant to others and society as a whole.

In assessing the psychosocial aspects of emotional health, it is important to evaluate the extent to which the person has a sense of identity and self-acceptance despite awareness of weaknesses. Emotional well-being is closely linked to developmental tasks for the various age-groups. Appropriate completion of the tasks increases one's positive attitude and acceptance of self and provides a basis for openness to new experiences, acceptance of others, and the foundation for progression to the next developmental task.

Emotional well-being is influenced by many factors. Some of the more important of these are the uniqueness of each individual, the environment and circumstances in which the person was raised and lives, the perceived role in family and community, and successful accomplishment of various developmental tasks throughout life.

As one progresses through the life cycle there are natural challenges and stresses relating to the establishment of life goals, family, and career. Success in meeting these challenges builds self-esteem, satisfaction, and skills for problem solving, all of which contribute to emotional well-being. Failure in meeting challenges leads to feelings of anxiety, stress, conflict, frustration, and hostility that detract from emotional well-being. If the client is anxious, it is important to determine the degree of anxiety involved, recognizing that mild anxiety can facilitate problem solving, whereas even moderate anxiety levels may decrease the ability of the individual to resolve problems as a means of decreasing stress. With high levels of anxiety, the individual may lose the ability to function and feel overwhelmed, totally unable to mobilize appropriate coping mechanisms that would decrease the stress level.

ADULT

To achieve an acceptable level of emotional health, the adult will seek to be at peace with self, others, and the environment. This requires one to develop an adequate sense of identity—that is, self-knowledge, self-understanding, and self-acceptance. Ideally, the adult can acknowledge his or her personal strengths and weaknesses; accept constructive criticism; postpone gratification of his or her needs; set goals; develop a value system; utilize past experiences in planning for the present and the future; take responsibility for his or her learning needs; obtain satisfaction from work; integrate cognition, emotion, and action; and resolve conflicts.

When relating to others, the emotionally healthy adult can develop and sustain mutually satisfying relationships; terminate harmful relationships; collaborate and compromise with others; communicate directly both verbally and nonverbally; communicate appropriately for the situation; and be respectful of others.

The healthy adult is able to organize and control his or her environment. In response to changes in the environment, the adult demonstrates adequate coping skills to adapt to the changes. The activities carried out by an emotionally healthy adult within the environment are planned, purposeful, and responsible. The adult who does not possess all of these characteristics is not necessarily mentally ill but may have less chance for optimum functioning. For instance, everyone experiences stress in daily life, but some individuals are better able to cope with it than others. Optimum stress is stress that allows the individual to maximize health and performance.

The individual will experience problems only if the life stress is either too great or too little to allow adjustment.

OLDER ADULT

A satisfactory emotional health status in the elderly requires adaptation to both internal and external changes. There are numerous physical changes related to the aging process that may make adaptation more difficult for the older person. Many of the changes, however, have psychosocial implications. These may include death of a spouse or decreased income to meet costs of living.

If the older person has adapted satisfactorily to changes in circumstances throughout life, the likelihood is that this process will continue to serve him or her well. If, however, the person has been somewhat rigid and lacked the ability to adapt as a younger person, the increasing requirement for adaptation with the aging process may be overwhelming. Generally, the older person who is optimistic and flexible is perceived to be emotionally healthy and fulfilled.

EXPECTANT PARENT

The nurse will assess both parents at the time of the first contact to determine attitudes and feelings about the pregnancy. These observations during the prenatal period can indicate possible areas for teaching, clarification, and planning to facilitate the entrance of a new baby into the family.

Pregnancy is an emotionally significant event in the life of the woman. Each woman must accomplish specific emotional tasks of pregnancy during each trimester. These tasks involve the mother's acceptance of the fetus as part of her body; then the fetus develops a separate identity; and finally the woman prepares for separation from the fetus. During pregnancy, many feelings emerge, ranging from joy to anxiety. The woman feels she is vulnerable and has feelings of dependency. She is eager to produce a normal, healthy baby. If this is her first child many fears occur. If she has had problems during the pregnancy, a perfect outcome may not be a reality.

In today's society, some women postpone childbearing until after 35 years of age. Women in this age-group who are beginning to have children will experience changes in life-style and developmental tasks. They may no longer have anything in common with friends who have older children. There are many questions to address—what will it be like at 50 to care for a 10-year-old? Will there be energy for the child-rearing years?

NEWBORN

The normal baby at birth is able to see, hear, smell, and feel. As the baby is able to focus on the parent's face, hear familiar voices, and feel the skin while being handled, the newborn begins the bonding process with the parents. To facilitate the emotional health of the newborn, it is the responsibility of the parent or care giver to be sensitive to these behaviors that help the newborn to interact with its new world.

An important aspect of creating and maintaining a sense of well-being for the newborn is to keep it closely swaddled. This produces a sense of close protection similar to that of the newborn's recent environment, the uterus. The tone of the newborn's cry will indicate its level of anxiety when the security of close wrapping is removed for any purpose.

Crying is the primary means of communication for the newborn. The appropriate parenting response to the baby's cry is to determine its need and meet it whether it is for food, clean clothing, or physical contact. There is little or no validity to the notion that picking up a child in response to crying will "spoil" it. Quite the contrary, newborns have an emotional need for cuddling, to feel the warmth and closeness of the parents.

INFANT/CHILD/ADOLESCENT

Meeting the developmental tasks of childhood appropriately facilitates positive mental well-being as an adult. The child's world is controlled by the care giver. Therefore, it is imperative that the care giver communicate freely and nonjudgmentally with the child to promote feelings of security, minimize tension, and help the child in fixing role identity. It may sometimes be difficult for parents to accept the behavior of the child because biases, culture, personal values, and anxiety can influence this acceptance. It is much easier for the parent to disapprove of unacceptable behavior than it is to accept the behavior and work toward modification of it. It is necessary to reassure the child that he or she is accepted, but that certain behaviors are not appropriate or acceptable.

During the developmental process, when the child's feelings are beginning to develop, he or she may become frustrated or resort to anger because of the surrounding situations. The child may even regress if a situation becomes too stressful. The parent can let the child know that these feelings are normal, but at the same time set limits on behaviors that are acceptable in expressing these angry feelings.

Limits are placed on various behaviors for all of us throughout life. Setting limits on a child's behavior allows the progression and exploration necessary to develop a sense of trust and security with the parent. An integral part of developing this sense of trust and security is the consistency with which the limits are applied.

The adolescent's conceptual world is starting to be filled with self and life. The adolescent is very self-centered, has difficulty accepting parental limits, and will frequently test the limits set. Parents need to be flexible in setting limits for the adolescent. Negotiation of certain limits between the parent and teenager is permissible. These might include curfew hours, clothing allowance or other areas of particular concern to the teenager. The parent, at this point, can retain control but be flexible in the limit setting, which will allow the adolescent to develop a sense of responsibility and enhance decision-making and communication skills.

The adolescent period is a time of high anxiety because of the psychological and physiological changes that take place. Sensitivity and skill are required to help the teenager deal with the strong inner feelings that may be manifested during these turbulent years of passage from childhood to adulthood. It may be difficult for parents to accept that the adolescent cannot discuss or chooses not to share feelings with them. This is the time for parents to encourage their child to discuss feelings with a responsible adult he or she feels comfortable talking to and who can be more objective.

QUESTIONNAIRE

ADULT

Do you feel you have control over your own life?

How would you describe yourself? (Consider casual, easygoing, competitive, rushed, taking things one at a time, slow in doing things, tolerating uncertainty, working all the time [even on vacation], optimistic, pessimistic.)

Do you hide your feelings, laugh at yourself, accept your good and bad aspects, accept others as they are, have empathy for how others feel?

Do you prefer to do things your way, stick to your principles no matter what, insist on full value for all purchases, like everything you do to be perfect, do things precisely to the last detail, get tense when your daily schedule is upset, plan time so as not to be late, make lists for your activities, strictly fulfill your obligations, get upset when you don't finish a task?

Are you critical of those who do not live up to your standards, upset by changes in environment or people, meticulous, fussy about possessions, bothered when surroundings are not clean, badly shaken if someone takes advantage of you?

Do you view your life as enjoyable? (Consider selective television watching, reading books, interests, pets, clubs/organizations.)

Do you take time and appreciate what life has to offer? (Consider ballet, theater, symphony, opera, museum, camping, fishing, hiking, going to a park, listening to the birds, smelling wild flowers, looking at the sky, stargazing, generally enjoying nature.)

How do you get along with people? (Consider worry more about how to present yourself to newcomers rather than how to treat them, fear of not being liked by others, enjoyment of playing, socializing with others.)

What are your thoughts like? (Consider wandering and rambling thoughts, lack of concentration, difficulty making decisions, slow or fast thinking, difficulty making people understand you.)

Do you feel you are flexible? (Consider variation, uniformity of activities, easily upset by unexpected events, things.)

Are you able to trust and value your own judgment, the decisions you make?

How do you solve your problems? (Consider alone, need others to help, avoidance.)

Does the way you solve your problems work for you?

What sort of things do you think about a lot? (Consider dwelling on one idea too much, difficulty getting asleep because of repetitive thoughts.)

Are you a "moody" person? (Consider frequent ups and downs, mild blue spells, related physical complaints, crying spells, feel like crying.)

How do you feel after you lose something or someone important to you? (Consider recent loss, how handled, ability to grieve, apathetic, detached, indifferent.)

What part of the day do you feel worst/best?

How do you feel about your life?

How do you feel about your job? (Consider likes, dislikes, stresses, rewards, challenges, time spent working on the job, at home, career changes.)

What kind of person would you say you are? Describe yourself.

Do you like yourself?

Are there changes you would like to make?

What do you think of your body? (Consider satisfaction, dissatisfaction, scars, loss of body parts.)

What was your life like when you were growing up?

Would you say you have reached or are reaching your life dreams and goals?

Has life been good to you?

How have you felt recently? (Consider depressed, anxious, lonely, stressed, guilty, bored, angry, resentful, fearful.)

What brought these feelings on?

What are you doing about them?

Is it helping?

Modifications for the Older Adult

How do you feel about getting older? (Consider feeling useless, unwanted, dependent, independent.)

How do you feel about retirement?

Has life become better or worse as you have aged? (Consider changes in income, health, living arrangements, friends, activities.)

Is being older the way you thought it would be? (Consider feelings, pleasures, satisfaction, dissatisfaction.)

Do you find time to reminisce? (Consider subject matter, diary, photo album, letters, mementos, souvenirs.)

Have you made any changes in your life to compensate for losses?

What are your feelings about death? (Consider self, significant others.)

What are your experiences with death or illness? (Consider self, close friends, spouse, other relatives or changes made to compensate for losses.)

Have you made arrangements for your death? (Consider funeral, living will, body donation to science, transplants, will.)

Do you live alone? If so, how long and what are your feelings about being alone?

Modifications for the Expectant Parent

Have you ever lost a baby? (Consider miscarriage [month], stillbirth, fetal demise, neonatal death.)

How do you feel about being pregnant? (Consider changes experienced during this time, number of other children.)

How does the father feel about this pregnancy?

What is your relationship with the father of this baby?

What is your relationship with your mother?

Do you feel you can depend on someone during your pregnancy?

What are your concerns or worries at this time?

Do you feel the baby is part of you?

At times do you feel you must protect yourself and the baby?

Tell me about your baby. (Consider what the baby will look like, gender, behavior, future plans for the baby.)

What things have you gotten for the baby?

What do you think labor will be like?

Modifications for the Newborn

How much time do you and the father spend holding your baby closely?

How do your other children interact with the baby?

How much time does your baby spend crying and what do you do about it?

Modifications for the Infant/Child/Adolescent

Do any of the following things concern you about your infant/child? (Consider eating, sleeping, getting along with other children, and adults, physical complaints, fears, worries, nervousness, thumb-sucking, restlessness, stress, overactivity, sexual problems, frequent daydreaming, temper tantrums, physical handicaps, misuse of drugs, excessive crying, lying, stealing, poor coordination, destructive behavior, school discipline problems, grades, bedwetting, poor bladder or bowel control, speech problem, moody, shy.)

What do you do about these concerns?

What do you consider good and bad behavior?

Do you discipline your infant/child/adolescent? (Consider types, consistency, response patterns, rules, explained rationale, rewards.)

For what reasons do your parents reward or punish you?

What does being good or bad mean to you?

What are the best things about your life?

What are some of the things you would like to change about your life?

What are your plans for the future and how will you achieve them?

BIBLIOGRAPHY

Barnard, K., & Erickson, M. L. *Teaching children with developmental problems: A family care approach.* St. Louis: Mosby, 1976.

Bortner, R. W. A short rating scale as a potential measure of patterning a behavior. *Journal of Chronic Disease,* 1969, 22, 87 -91.

Butler, R., & Lewis, M. I. *Aging and mental health.* St. Louis: Mosby, 1982.

Cox, C. L. Motivation: Vehicle for public health nursing intervention? *Public Health Nursing,* 1985, 2(4), 202–212.

Cramer, L. *Freedom from compulsion.* New York: Simon & Schuster, 1976.

Department of Health Education. *Lifestyle assessment questionnaire.* Stevens Point, Wis.: University of Wisconsin, 1978.

Flavell, J. H. *The developmental psychology of Jean Piaget.* New York: Van Nostrand Reinhold, 1963.

Francis, G., & Munjas, B. *Manual of socialpsychologic assessment.* New York: Appleton-Century-Crofts, 1976.
Korner, A. F. Individual differences at birth; implications for early experience and later development. *American Journal of Orthopsychiatry,* 1974, *41*(4), 608–619.
Kozier, B., & Erb, G. *Fundamentals of nursing.* Menlo Park, Calif.: Addison-Wesley, 1983.
Kreigh, H. Z., & Perko, J. D. *Psychiatric and mental health nursing: Commitment to care and concern.* Reston, Va.: Reston Publishing, 1979.
Lawton, M. P., & Brody, E. Assessment of elder people: self-maintaining and instrumental activities of daily living. *Gerontologist,* 1969, *9,* 179–186.
McClelland, K. A. Self-conception and life satisfaction: Integrating aged subculture and activity theory. *Journal of Gerontology,* 1982, *37*(6), 723–732.
Newman, M. A., & Gaudiano, J. K. Depression as an explanation for decreased subjective time in the elderly. *Nursing Research,* 1984, *33*(3), 137–139.
Pender, N. J. *Health promotion in nursing practice* (2nd ed.). Norwalk, Conn.: Appleton & Lange, 1987.
Rahe, R. H., McKean, J. Jr., Arthur, K. J. A longitudinal study of life-change and illness patterns. *Journal of Psychosomatic Research,* 1967, *10,* 355–366.
Rainwater, A. J. Elderly loneliness and its relation to residential care. *Journal of Gerontological Nursing,* 1980, *6*(10), 593–599.
Roberts, C. S., & Feetham, S. L. Assessing family functioning across three areas of relationships. *Nursing Research,* 1982, *31*(4), 231–235.
Selye, H. Introduction. In Wheatley, D. (Ed.), *Stress and the heart.* New York: Raven Press, 1977.
Snow, R., & Crado, L. Emotional bondedness, subjective well-being, and health in elderly medical patients. *Journal of Gerontology,* 1982, *37*(5), 609–615.
Sorochan, W. D. *Personal health appraisal.* New York: Wiley, 1976.
Thompson, J., & Bowers, A. *Clinical manual of health assessment.* St. Louis: Mosby, 1980.
Wilson, H. S., & Kneisl, C. R. *Psychiatric nursing.* Menlo Park, Calif.: Addison-Wesley, 1979.
Wolff, L., Weitzel, M., Zornow, R. A., & Zsohar, H. *Fundamentals of nursing.* Philadelphia: Lippincott, 1983.
Zung, W. K. A self-rating depression scale. *Archives of General Psychiatry,* 1965, *12,* 63–70.

UNIT 9
Spirituality

INTRODUCTION

Some aspect of spirituality has been with us since the beginning of time. Many people's spiritual beliefs have evolved from the concepts of good and evil. Good deeds are rewarded, while evil is punished by an entity who is separate from the individual. The incorporation of these basic beliefs, concepts, and principles forms the basis for religious and spiritual systems.

Assessing the spiritual beliefs of an individual client is necessary to plan nursing care that will meet the client's spiritual needs. The need for the person to believe in a power higher than humankind is thought to be a universal one and is the basis for hope. With hope, the client can believe that the future will be better, and this frequently plays a significant role in the client's belief about health and illness.

It is important to recognize that spiritual beliefs may or may not be associated with religion. A religion is usually based on a formalized set of spiritual beliefs around which certain rituals are organized. The religion-based belief systems of many individuals give organization to the psychosocial components of their total health. The client may not belong to an organized religion, but still hold deep spiritual values that are important to assess and incorporate into a total healthcare plan. From time to time, the nurse will have clients who are agnostics or atheists who do not share in the majority's belief in a higher spiritual being. In this case, it is important that the nurse remain nonjudgmental while working with this client.

Religious practices do have a bearing on nursing care planning. For example, some religions place limitations on birth control practices and circumcision of male babies, or observe dietary restrictions. Spiritual practices may also have a bearing on the kind and type of health care that is sought by an individual. Because of their religious beliefs and values, some clients will refuse to have medications or blood products as part of their health and healing regimen.

There are many religions over the world and each of these may have several sects so that an in-depth understanding of these many belief systems is virtually impossible for the nurse. Some understanding of the principle tenets held by the major religions of the world will offer guidance to the nurse in assessing and planning client care.

Because spiritual values also have a cultural component, it is necessary to complete a cultural assessment to have a more well-rounded view of client needs. As with other parts of the assessment, the meaning and significance of a client's spiritual and cultural values may be more readily assessed through a sensitive discussion of matters of concern rather than asking many questions. Knowledge of the spiritual belief will allow the nurse to plan care that will meet these varying needs of clients and generally facilitate the healing process.

ADULT

The adult uses rituals and traditions to give meaning and significance to life. Nurturing children often allows the adult to analyze many of his or her values, including beliefs about spirituality. The adult may find that the religious education received as a child will help to answer the difficult questions his or her children may pose in developing their spiritual values.

The maturing adult may attempt to bridge any differences between inner self and religion through interpersonal relationships. Spiritual development and maturity require an integration of wisdom, morality, ethics, hope, and compassion. Spiritual development pulls together the adult's total developmental process and carries him or her into the final portion of life.

OLDER ADULT

The mature individual is able to incorporate life experiences into spiritual development so that it is part of the total development process. As a person ages, this incorporation, along with development in other dimensions, brings him or her to a higher level of individuality, organization, and differentiation. The spiritual component of aging allows development of a philosophy of life and peace with one's place in the world as well as peace with relationships with family and others. Some evaluation of where the older person is in this process will facilitate appropriate nursing care planning.

EXPECTANT PARENT

The influence of other individuals, especially within the family, plays an important part in the development and maintenance of one's spirituality. An individual's concept of religion governs that individual's behavior and the behavior expected from others. Each religious group has its own value for childbearing and child-rearing practices. There are rituals, rules, and procedures. Abortion, premarital sex, divorce, adultery, and the number of children may be some issues discussed within a spiritual group. The impact of religion on the couple will also affect the life of the child.

The expectant mother often feels vulnerable during her pregnancy and fears that something may endanger her baby. It is the concept of hope as an aspect of spirituality that assists her to manage her fears regarding her unborn child. The belief that she will have a healthy baby helps the mother to cope with the more uncomfortable aspects of her pregnancy.

NEWBORN

Activities related to spirituality in the newborn are based on the belief system of the parents. During the newborn period, there may be many religious rituals performed that also have cultural foundations. There may be godparents who choose the baby's name, or a grandparent who presents the child to the extended family, or a baptism before the baby is 3 months old, or the rite of circumcision performed on the eighth day. These rituals are important to the parents, their families, and often the community at large. The nurse should begin to develop an understanding of the role that spirituality plays in many of the aspects of the parent–newborn cycle, because many of these religious practices have a direct influence upon the life of the child.

INFANT/CHILD/ADOLESCENT

The toddler begins to understand spirituality by imitating the spiritual behavior of its parents. During the preschool years, the child begins to develop a sense of right and wrong and asks questions about religion. The child believes that God is responsible for physical phenomena that occur in the environment, such as wind and rain.

A greater understanding of right and wrong further develops during the school-age years. The child expects rewards for good behavior and punishment for bad behavior. The child, when he or she prays, believes that the prayers will be answered. In time, the child realizes that prayers are not always answered as they are petitioned. The child also does not accept religion blindly but is now beginning to raise questions regarding spirituality.

The adolescent analyzes religion from the points of view of the parents and others, as well as science. This analysis assists the teenager in the choice of accepting his or her parents' spirituality or developing an independent value system. A strong belief system can give the adolescent strength during developmental crises.

QUESTIONNAIRE

ADULT

Is there a spiritual belief system that is important to you? (Consider components, meaning, help to you, how.)

Are any practices within this belief system particularly important to you? (Consider what they are [prayer, books, symbols, attendance], how are they used.)

Is your spiritual belief system organized around a specific denomination, organization, church?

If so, which one, and how actively are you involved?

Do other family members belong to the same organization?

If not, does this cause any problems?

Who is the most important person to you?

To whom do you turn when in need of help?

Is help generally available from this source?

In what ways do you receive help from this source?

What are your beliefs about the causes of disease, illness, and death?

Does your spiritual system help when you are not feeling well?

Does it influence health-care decisions in any way?

Are there any health treatments or dietary restrictions related to your beliefs?

Do you expect any spiritually related experiences from health or health-related activities?

Do you relate religion to good health in any way?

Have you ever engaged in faith healing?

Is prayer a part of your belief system?

How often do you pray, when, and with what results?

Does your spiritual belief system include a deity, such as God?

How does this entity function in your life?

In what ways are you helped with carrying out your faith?

Modifications for the Older Adult

Has your spiritual or religious belief system changed with age?

Do your spiritual or religious values mean any more or less to you as you age?

Are you able to carry out practices or rituals that meet your spiritual or religious needs? (Consider health, transportation, finances.) Has there been any difficulty in treating illness because of religious beliefs?

Modifications for the Expectant Parent

What will be the influence of spirituality or religion on your baby?

Does your pregnancy affect your religious practices in any way?

Are there any problems with pregnancy as a result of the spiritual belief system that you hold?

Modifications for the Newborn

What religious practices and rituals do you observe for the infant? (Consider circumcision, baptism, naming.)

Modifications for the Infant/Child/Adolescent

How old do you think a child is when the concepts of right and wrong will be understood?

Does your child ask questions about religious topics? (Consider heaven, hell, good, bad.)

How are religious or spiritual values taught within your family?

What does religion mean to you? (Consider prayers, church attendance, practices.)

BIBLIOGRAPHY

Burkhart, M. A. Dealing with spiritual concerns of clients in the community. *Journal of Community Health Nursing*, 1985, 2(4), 191–198.

Burnside, I. M., Ebersole, P., & Honea, H. E. *Psychosocial caring throughout the life span*. New York: McGraw-Hill, 1979.

Gress, D. S., & Bahr, R. *The aging person: A holistic perspective*. St. Louis: Mosby, 1984.

Kozier, B., & Erb, G. *Fundamentals of nursing*. Menlo Park, Calif.: Addison-Wesley, 1983.

Markides, R. S. Aging, religiosity, and adjustment longitudinal analysis. *Journal of Gerontology*, 1983, *38*(5), 621–625.

Narrow, B., & Buschle, K. *Fundamentals of nursing*. New York: Wiley, 1982.
Stoll, R. Guidelines for spiritual assessment. *American Journal of Nursing*, 1979, *79*, 1574–1579.
Thompson, J., & Bowers, A. *Clinical manual of health assessment*. St. Louis: Mosby, 1980.

UNIT 10

Interpersonal Relationships

INTRODUCTION

Interpersonal relationships are those interactions an individual has with other persons and groups. To establish interpersonal relationships, one first needs to feel comfortable with oneself. The individual who knows his or her "good" and "bad" points and is able to live with them is able to develop closer relationships with others. The development of a close or intimate contact with a significant other involves the establishment of a give-and-take relationship so it will be mutally satisfying. Sometimes, one person will need to assume more responsibility within the relationship than the other. For example, in the parent–child relationship, the parent, not the child, is responsible for the relationship or, in the nurse–client relationship, the nurse assumes more responsibility when the client is ill.

Group interpersonal relationships are formed to achieve various goals. These might include communication among family members toward achievement of family objectives; maintenance of cultural traditions, as in a religious activity; or development of satisfactory working conditions, as in an office. These types of relationships allow individuals to develop a sense of belonging within their social, cultural, and economic environments.

An analysis of the various roles played by each person in interpersonal relationships allows understanding of how one, as an individual, functions within society. A role is composed of certain behaviors and functions performed by a person occupying a given position in society. Each person can enact roles differently; however, there are certain rights, duties, obligations, and privileges or role expectations that tell how one should perform a role. The way one performs one's role and the importance attached to it influences interpersonal relationships. The number of roles a person has to perform, how involved the person is in the role, the amount of time spent in the role, how the individual feels about being in the role, and the knowledge the person has about the role affect role performance. Incongruity among one or all of these factors can be a source of conflict. If all of these factors interact smoothly, the performer will be in agreement or in harmony with the role.

ADULT

The young adult years are usually very productive, but many changes occur at this time in life. The young adult may be expected to be a wife or husband, mother or father, sister or brother, and breadwinner. The expectations for each of these roles may be legitimate but impossible to fulfill. Other people who hold the individual to these expectations may be unaware of the other expectations. The nurse may assist the young adult to identify, prevent, or cope with potential conflict among the roles; set priorities for each role; analyze feelings regarding certain roles; identify ways to decrease the importance of and time spent in some of the roles; and develop communication strategies to gain more information about the roles. Assisting the client to clarify roles will allow time to develop one-to-one and group interpersonal relationships.

The years between the ages of 35 to 65 are spent building and maintaining the society. The major role of the middle adult is a contributory one. There are usually few role problems during these years, and this is a consistent and productive time in the individual's life. Problems experienced with roles and interpersonal relationships are usually caused by situational factors. There could be role conflict within the marriage relationship or lack of satisfaction with job or career changes.

OLDER ADULT

Interpersonal relationships in the elderly are dependent, to a great extent, on the person's ability to adapt to new or different roles. Role development for older persons may lead toward lesser levels of privilege and responsibility. This decreased responsibility is perhaps more easily seen in the male's role as breadwinner and family provider, a work-related role. If the other roles in his life are based primarily on his status as an employed person, then with retirement will come changes in many of the person's interpersonal relationships. An example of this would be a blue-collar worker who, in addition to his role in industry, is also a union steward and captain of one of the company baseball teams. Retirement from the job, therefore, means multiple adjustments in roles and alterations of interpersonal relationships at several levels.

Frequently, changes in roles and interpersonal relationships are more predictable for men than for women. This would be particularly true for the woman who has not worked or does not work outside the home. The man may know, years ahead of time, that he will be retiring at a certain age and, theoretically, at least, should be able to plan toward that time.

The woman, however, has little opportunity to plan for the effect that the death of her husband will have on her role. Suddenly, with no one to cook, launder, and keep house for, her role as housewife will simply disappear. The woman may not know ahead of time when her last child will leave home, when menopause will relieve her of the problem of birth control, or when she may become a grandmother. Reason tells us that definition of new roles and changes in interpersonal relationships should be eased when alterations are predefined rather than unpredictable. The older person, however, is undergoing a series of changes requiring adaptation. If the client becomes overwhelmed by the process and is unable to adapt, interpersonal relationships will suffer.

One typically pleasant new role or interpersonal relationship associated with older persons is that of grandparenthood. Generally this is seen as a positive aspect of this portion of the life cycle. Interpersonal relationships between children and their grandparents are frequently defined by cultural factors and may range from the grandparent being elder and teacher to being provider and resource person. The mobile society of today frequently puts long distances between families, and children may be deprived of close relationships with one or both sets of grandparents. However, if the older person has made a fairly satisfactory adjustment to the aging process and related new roles, grandparenthood can be a wonderful time of enjoyment for all involved.

EXPECTANT PARENT

There are many factors that determine a woman's or man's readiness to take on the role of mother or father. The couple must have a combination of emotional maturity, the desire to have a baby, and establish that the child will be a value to them. The role of parenting, however, may present conflict to the couple. The birth of a child carries with it a sense of responsibility. If role expectation of the new parent is not explicit, different interpretations arise, leading to uncertainty as to what is expected. In our society, it is difficult for couples to learn parenting skills. We no longer have large families, and children do not have the opportunity to care for many brothers and sisters. Divorce also disrupts many families, and often they are separated by many miles from extended family members. A new mother, if she is fortunate, has her mother come for a week or two after she has her baby. It is during this time that the new grandmother teaches the new mother how to care for the new baby.

Measures can be employed to reduce conflicts in role expectations. If the new parent tries a particular technique with the new baby and it works, this reduces some conflict and role strain. The social reinforcement from significant others can also reduce new role conflict. The nurse can provide additional support in helping the new parents function appropriately in their parenting role.

NEWBORN

Much has been written about mother–infant bonding or attachment. When a new mother sees her newborn, love can occur in various degrees. This relationship can be love at first sight or can occur in various stages as it grows over time. Bonding that occurs over a longer time and is based on strong attachment is crucial to the survival and development of the child. Inadequate bonding may contribute to developmental problems for the child, and if this is thought to be a problem it must be carefully assessed to determine the underlying cause. This is especially true for the mother who has had a cesarean birth. The mother may need time to reflect on the birth of her child and to assimilate her new role. This will include time for sleep, rest, and discussion of the labor and delivery. Meeting these components of the mother's needs will facilitate a love relationship as it develops between mother and baby.

INFANT/CHILD/ADOLESCENT

The roles learned during the pediatric years are preparatory in nature. The child is learning to perform in expected ways that are consistent with position in the family and culture. The child begins to learn to interact with others on a one-to-one basis through contacts with peers in school, play, and other social situations.

A child usually does not experience role conflict, but there are familial factors that can influence the child's ability to relate to other people. These may include family size, sibling position, sex, whether or not the mother is employed outside the home, and whether or not the father is absent as a result of divorce or extensive travel.

Numerous other factors influence the child's interpersonal relationships and performance of roles. Adjustments must be made by the child if handicapped or chronically ill, if a sibling or parent dies, and if a stepparent and stepsiblings enter his or her life.

One of the tasks of the adolescent years is role refinement. Much energy is expended to define "who I am" and "where I am going." This often results in role conflict and role overload. This affects the interpersonal interaction between self, peers, and family members.

QUESTIONNAIRE

ADULT

Describe each of your family members. (Consider age of parents, how their age has affected client's relationship with them.)

Where do family members live?

Do you get together as a family often? (Consider family closeness, togetherness, family view of each other.)

What roles do your family members have? (Consider jobs of various members within the family, are family members comfortable in these roles and jobs, amount of time spent with family.)

What is the central concern within your family and are there difficulties that interfere with it?

Are there family members or friends who will help you and, if so, how do they help?

Are your physical and emotional needs met by your family?

Are family experiences broad or narrow?

Do you feel you can cope with difficulties? (Consider crucial or decisive situations in life and how well they were handled.)

What topics are hardest to talk about within the family? (Consider problems and issues being discussed, verbal and nonverbal communication, clarity of communication within the family.)

In your family are there goals toward which each member works?

Do you feel free to pursue a goal with which the family is in disagreement?

Does the family see itself as sick or healthy?

Describe your work or occupation. (Consider job rotation or split shifts, working on weekends, working at more than one job, number of hours of work per week, job satisfaction, career choice.)

How long have you been at this job? (Consider opportunity for advancement.)

Do you like the work you do and get along with other employees?

What does your family think about your occupation?

Are you unemployed? (Consider why not working, satisfaction with not working, kinds of jobs held, why left.)

Have you served in the military? (Consider for how long, branch of service, highest rank, job done.)

How many years of schooling have you completed?

Are you attending any educational program now? If so, describe.

Are you satisfied with your education? (Consider comparison with other members of family; if different, does it cause any problems?)

When did you first leave home? (Consider why, first living arrangements, major relationship during that time, any difficulties with giving, sharing.)

When did you meet your spouse? (Consider how, what was attraction, is it still there, decision to marry, who suggested, what was response.)

Has your spouse been married before? (Consider children from previous marriage, obstacles or problems surrounding marriage earlier or now, resolution to problems, expectations of one another.)

How is your relationship with your spouse?

Are your plans working out? (Consider ability to resolve disagreements, how you get along with in-laws.)

Do you have children as a result of this marriage? (Consider beliefs about raising children, how implemented, problems with child rearing, satisfaction with the way they are turning out.)

If not married, are you involved in an intimate relationship? (Consider person, relationship, commitment to this person, the meaning of the person to you.)

If divorced, how does your previous marriage affect your present relationship?

Describe a typical day.

What is the greatest accomplishment in life to date?

What major events have occurred in last five years? (Consider death, divorce, illness, legal problems, marriage, job loss.)

Are you satisfied with your life? (Consider leisure time, social life, life-style, living arrangements, family situations and relationships, sex life, finances, job, education, health, religious activities, political-civic-volunteer work, yourself.)

Are you comfortable making new friends and acquaintances? (Consider speaking to strangers, touching others, being touched by others.)

Modifications for the Older Adult

What is your relationship with your children or grandchildren?

How has the state of physical health affected you and your spouse? (Consider life-style, finances, adjustments.)

Has your role within the family changed with aging?

Do you feel free to ask assistance of family and friends to accomplish tasks you are no longer able to do?

Is there a family support system to assist with handling the deaths of family members and cohorts? (Consider reaction to deaths of parents, friends.)

Is your spouse living? (Consider satisfaction with the closeness and sharing; If no, consider reaction to death of spouse, a new partner, satisfactory relationship.)

What are your thoughts and plans for the future?

Modifications for the Expectant Parent

How do you feel about being pregnant? (Consider unplanned or planned pregnancy, job, income, status, losses, role.)

How does the father feel about the pregnancy?

As a child was there someone in your immediate family who you saw as a kind and loving person? (Consider most loving person, what parents are like.)

Do you feel you will need help when you get home from the hospital? (Consider plans, expectations.)

Is there someone to help you when you get home?

Who will help take over some of your household tasks when you bring the baby home?

How do you expect the baby to change your life?

How do you feel about your baby's appearance? (Consider behavior, care for self, baby at home.)

Do you and/or your partner have any thoughts and ideas on changing life-styles? (Consider working hours, home adjustments pertaining to pregnancy, new baby, siblings.)

Modifications for the Newborn

Observations to be made by the nurse:

Does mother verbalize to infant, touch, pick up?

Once infant is picked up, does mother stroke, caress, rock, or talk to infant while holding?

Is there eye contact, face-to-face contact?

How near to the infant is mother when making sounds?

Does infant's activity change in response to sounds?

Does infant make sounds and how often?

At what point in fussing or crying does mother respond to infant?

Does the mother understand infant cries?

If infant does not respond to mother's efforts, what is her response?

Modifications for the Infant/Child/Adolescent

How has the infant changed your life?

What school is child attending?

What grade are you in?

How are you doing with your studies and other interests?

How do you feel about yourself? (Consider shy, outgoing.)

Do you make friends easily and how many friends do you have?

What clubs and activities do you participate in?

What do you want to be when you grow up?

Do you usually agree or disagree with your family, friends and teachers?

When you get angry what do you do?

What are parents' attitudes toward the things you do? (Consider accepting, permissive, controlling, demanding.)

How do you feel about your parents and other adults? (Consider compliant, defiant, rebellious, assertive.)

What do you think your parents feel about your work at school, your friends, other activities? (Consider satisfaction with these things.)

How do you feel about this?

BIBLIOGRAPHY

Fields, W., & McGinn-Campbell, K. *Introduction to health assessment*. Reston, Va.: Reston Publishing, 1983.

Francis, G., & Munjas, B. *Manual of socialpsychologic assessment*. New York: Appleton-Century-Crofts, 1976.

Funke-Furber, J. *Reliability and validity testing of maternal adaptive behavior*. Edmonton, Alb.: University of Alberta, Faculty of Nursing, 1978.

Green, C. P. How to recognize hostility and what to do about it. *American Journal of Nursing*, 1986, *86*(11), 230–234.

Kreigh, H., & Perko, J. *Psychiatric and mental health nursing: Commitment to care and concern*. Reston, Va.: Reston Publishing, 1984.

Lynam, M. J. Adolescent communication: Understanding its dynamics and factoring its development. *Nursing Papers*, 1986, *18*(1), 67–77.

Powell, M. L., & Pipes, P. L. *Assessment and management of developmental changes and problems in children*. St. Louis: Mosby, 1981.

Reiser, S. A tool to facilitate mother-infant attachment. *Nursing Journal of Obstetric, Gynecologic, and Neonatal Nursing*, 1981, *10*, 294–296.

Whaley, L., & Wong, D. *Nursing care of infants and children*. St. Louis: Mosby, 1983.

UNIT 11
Sexuality

INTRODUCTION

Sexual behavior is a part of life from puberty to very old age, though there may be declines of function with aging. Developmental theorists indicate that sex-role identification begins by age three. Sex-role identification as part of human sexuality is influenced greatly by family and cultural values. Families with very traditional cultural values will expect children to identify strongly with the parent of the same sex. Many contemporary American families are redefining roles and values, which may have a profound effect on the future role-identification processes of the offspring. Children of both sexes are being treated more equally so that, it is hoped, the female child will no longer have the stereotyped limitations in role development that were once commonplace.

The sexual identity that is established in early childhood becomes a significant force during the adolescent years. Even with the many changes in values related to sexuality, much of the learning about sexual function and other related matters may be repressed or suppressed. This is usually done inadvertently by parents or families in their effort to direct expression of their child's sexual feelings and activities into socially acceptable channels. Lack of information about sexual function and our limited sex education programs in schools bring adolescents into adulthood with varying levels of knowledge and understanding of human sexuality.

With some knowledge, some impulsivity, and some autonomous behavior, the young adult enters into the period of life that will ultimately produce another generation to begin the cycle again. Preparation for this role has, traditionally, been marginal. The influences of the women's liberation movement, and the gay rights activists, and greater acceptance of divorce, cohabitation, and premarital sex may confuse the young person. The young adult must define role and personal values, incorporate family and cultural influences, and make choices carefully to develop a successful long-term relationship.

Sexual expression in the later years may take a different form of expression as bodily functions decline and women outnumber men, but throughout life, sex and sexuality should be pleasurable. Expression of these basic human needs should be rewarding and fulfilling.

As one assesses human sexuality it is important to recognize the complexity of the construct. Each of us brings our infant and childhood experiences, which have been shaped and defined by families, teachers, societal values, and ourselves. Some of these are positive, others negative, and many influences are beyond our awareness. Assisting a client with sorting out potential problems in this part of psychosocial assessment requires patience, understanding, and sensitivity on the part of the nurse in exploring this very private function.

Quite often the sexual history is not completed by the health-care professional because of a discomfort with the subject or inexperience with the appropriate data to be gathered. There are two ways in which the health-care provider can become comfortable with assessment of sexual health. Analysis of one's own feelings about sexual health is the first step. The second step is to establish a therapeutic relationship with the client before gathering data in this area.

ADULT

The tasks of sexual development for the adult are numerous. As one proceeds along the developmental continuum from the young adult years to the middle adult years the developmental tasks change. The young adult is expected to establish an involved, mutual, and reciprocal physiological and psychological intimacy with another person. He or she learns to give and receive love. Consolidation of the union and rearing children take place during the adult years. Developing a newly satisfying relationship with a partner is necessary during the middle years, when the children leave home.

The meaning and value an adult places upon sexuality is dependent upon the interrelationship of physical, mental, emotional, psychological, social, and spiritual abilities. For example, the woman who is experiencing menopause may have vaginal dryness and thinning secondary to hormonal changes. Emotionally she may be depressed and upset because of the loss of spontaneity in her sex life caused by the necessity of preparations to assist in intercourse. On the other hand, she may discover a new enjoyment of sex, now that the fear of pregnancy is eliminated.

The purpose of sexuality during the adult years is reproduction and giving and receiving physical and psychological pleasure. Many myths surround adult sexuality, including the following: young adults want and have sex more often than older adults; sexual capability is stronger during the young adult years than during the older adult years; middle adults have more sexual knowledge and skill than younger adults; and adult females have limited desire, knowledge, skill, and physical capability for sexual relationships. With regard to sexual matters, our attitudes change slowly.

OLDER ADULT

In assessing sexual functioning for the older person, one must recognize the myths, misconceptions, and stereotypes associated with this age-group. The literature refers to the concept of sexless old age assumed by our society. The idea that one might live out one's later years without sexual contact is perhaps based on several factors. There are physiological changes that are part of the aging process. These include such things as menopause and thinning vaginal walls in women. For men there is a gradual slowing of erection time, decrease in the firmness of the erection, and decreased volume of ejaculate. Age-related physiological changes often cause the older person to have increased anxiety about maintaining sexual function. It is important that an adequate assessment be made of the sexual functioning of the older person and appropriate guidance and teaching be offered. Otherwise, the continuing physiological changes may cause increased mental distress, and the decline becomes a self-fulfilling prophecy. Understanding by the older person of the sexual changes as they progress allows adaptation and decreased anxiety, which facilitates sexual functioning.

Perhaps one of the most important factors in maintaining sexual functioning for older persons is the availability of a suitable partner.

A patient, loving person can assist a partner toward a fuller enjoyment of sexual contact. However, women outlive men by an average of seven years. In addition, the husband is usually older at the time of marriage. Therefore, there are several years in the life of an average older woman in which she may have to seek alternate means of sexual expression.

Exploration of sexuality and sexual values of any client can be difficult for the nurse but is perhaps most problematical with the older person. Most have lived lives in which sexual matters were not discussed. Security about one's own sexuality and a nonjudgmental attitude toward the client are essential for the nurse as the assessment of sexual functioning in the older person is made.

EXPECTANT PARENT

Until recently, sex during pregnancy was an undiscussed subject. It is now known that sexual desires and responses are as individual as each woman. Some feel that pregnancy allows for an openness and less fear, and orgasm intensifies. Other women feel that their responses decrease and they lose their sex drive.

There are still many fears and cultural taboos associated with coitus during pregnancy. Many believe that intercourse will harm the fetus or begin labor. Fulfillment of sexual needs does not have to terminate just because a woman is pregnant. Love can be shared in touch and caress. Caring, being loved, feeling important and attractive to her mate is important for the woman. If her protruding abdomen makes her feel fat and unattractive she may believe her mate does not find her sexually attractive during pregnancy. The woman needs reassurance, support, and love.

Different sexual patterns may need to be established during pregnancy, since sexual positions may not be as comfortable because of the increased uterine size. The nurse needs to assess each couple regarding their sexuality and help them decide what is best for them based on their needs, desires, and belief patterns.

The doctor often instructs the client not to put anything into the vagina for six weeks after delivery. This truly is not realistic. Generally, coitus may resume when the woman feels she is ready or when the bleeding stops. Many women have episiotomies or even lacerations and may fear resuming intercourse. These issues need to be discussed with the woman after delivery. Caring for a new baby may also require most of her energy and there may not be enough energy left for sexual activities with her mate. Coitus is not the only way to release sexual tension, and the measures of touch and masturbation need to be discussed with the couple.

NEWBORN

In female newborns, the vulva is edematous and the clitoris is prominent because of maternal hormone stimulation. Some female babies may even have enlarged breast tissue and have a scant bloody vaginal discharge. This results from absorption of the sex hormones from the mother before birth.

The scrotum of male newborns may be edematous because of birth trauma. If the baby is circumcised, the glans is sore and red. The foreskin of uncircumcised males is not retractable until age three to four and often not until puberty. The parents may have questions about physical manifestations in the newborns. These are real concerns and must be addressed by the nurse. Such questions need to be resolved for the child's sake.

INFANT/CHILD/ADOLESCENT

A new openness regarding sexuality developed in this country during the 1960s and 1970s. Children of all ages are more aware of sexuality and require information and assistance to develop a clear picture of themselves as sexual human beings. Sexuality is a complex human function that is developed as a result of the intermeshing of the physical, mental, emotional, social, and spiritual development of the individual. All of these dimensions influence how the person will react to sexual education and how he or she will utilize the teaching. Because these variables are dynamic, it is important to note that individuals of all ages may require sex education, not just children.

Touch is extremely important for sexual development during the infant years. As the care giver cuddles and hugs the infant, the baby learns to feel good about its body. The infant also learns that this type of stimulus causes a pleasant body response. The infant then learns that self-stimulation of the body, including the genitalia, is pleasurable. It may be difficult for the care giver to understand that infant self-stimulation is not detrimental. This is because adults often compare this purely physical phenomenon with adult sexuality, which has emotional, psychological, and sociocultural overtones. Education at this time is directed toward helping the parents learn about the normal development of their infant.

During the childhood years an interest in and a curiosity about sexual development is common. At this age, children benefit from appropriate household nudity. It teaches them to be proud of their bodies and gives them the opportunity to ask questions regarding their sexuality in a nonthreatening environment. As the child gets older, privacy will become important, and this need should be respected by others in the household. This would be an appropriate time to discontinue the openness about nudity. The inquisitive nature of the child often leads to playing games such as "doctor" with children of the opposite sex. Children of the opposite sex may be so curious about each other's bodies that they may play "If you show me your body, I'll show you mine." The nurse needs to educate the care giver to recognize that the child does these things to explore and learn. The care giver needs to take this opportunity to educate the child about sexuality. If alarm, anger or anxiety is the response to these episodes, the child may begin to think that bodies—one's own or others'—are bad or dirty.

Appropriate sex education for the child includes an honest and open discussion of sexual development and the reproductive process. Children need to learn about conception, pregnancy, the birth process, menstruation, masturbation, and nocturnal emissions. This will help to ease the transition from childhood to adolescence. If the child is unaware that these are common aspects of sexual development he or she may become anxious and upset. The care giver may also require some education about these topics to be able to let the child know that the child's experiences and feelings are understood. The care giver's understanding will help the child to begin accepting his or her body and sexuality. Accepting one's own body and sexuality is essential to sexual fulfillment as an adult.

The adolescent period is a time of profound change in all aspects of a person's development. Puberty brings on bodily changes, and these changes lead to strong emotional upheaval. The body that once was comfortable and predictable changes suddenly. The most significant aspect of this change is the fact that adolescents have no control over these physical changes that impact on their sexuality and interpersonal relationships. Teenagers begin to assess their bodies critically. They may question the normality of their development, comparing the development of their genitalia with that of others. It is difficult for them to understand that they may develop at a different pace from their peers. Faster or slower physical development leads to anxiety for the teenager.

During the preadolescent years a sense of male or female identity develops. Initially the preteen seems to prefer relationships with others of the same sex. This is the time when strong best-friend relationships are formed. Next, teens begin socializing in mixed groups and finally progress to dates with a member of the opposite sex. At this time the teen may experience "growing pains," feel confused, alone, exposed, and worry about being different from peers with regard to this psychosocial development.

The adolescent establishes him- or herself as a sexually and socially independent person. To do this requires redefining the self within the context of a new body and new social environment. A lot of soul-searching and self-analysis go on in the attempt to determine an identity and values for many things. The teen tries to integrate parental values regarding sexuality with those of society. Although the teenager may rebel against parental values, usually the sexual values developed are congruent with, but independent of, those of the parents.

Education of the teen during these very vulnerable years is essential to the development of a healthy sexual attitude. The adolescent needs information about pregnancy and contraception, masturbation, homosexual encounters, nocturnal emissions, menstruation, body image, and sexual feelings. The teenager needs to know that these things are a common part of adolescent development This will equip him or her with the resources to cope with the changes and feelings experienced during this period. The adolescent also needs to know that there is nothing wrong with being different from one's peers in terms of sexual activity. Sexual activity should not begin until it is right for the individual. If a teenager becomes sexually active before acceptance of self as being responsible for the consequences of one's own actions, an unwanted pregnancy may result. Sexual activity among teens increases every year. Teens who have had sexual education are more likely to act responsibly in sexual encounters rather than be carried away by their emotions. Nurses need to accept opportunities to educate parents and other adults about the way teens develop a sense of responsibility for sexual activity so that resistance to sex education in the schools will decrease.

QUESTIONNAIRE

ADULT

Do you and your sexual partner agree on the frequency and nature of your sexual activities?

If married, are you sexually attracted to persons other than your spouse?

Does it cause problems?

Do you engage in sexual activities with more than one person?

How do you feel about seeking help for a sexual problem?

What method of birth control do you use?

Do you have difficulty communicating with someone of the opposite sex?

Is there anything you think your child needs to or wants to know that you are unable to discuss with him or her?

Would you like help from someone in discussing that difficult area?

Who was most influential in teaching you about sex and how to be a man (woman)?

What were your early beliefs and attitudes about sex? In what way are your beliefs and attitudes different now?

When was your first period?

Do you recall masturbating? (Consider feelings about it.)

Have you had any homosexual experiences?

Have you had heterosexual, homosexual, or bisexual experiences from which you feel at risk for AIDS?

How often do you awaken with an erection during the night or in the morning?

Are you familiar with any other words for intercourse?

How do you see yourself as a man (woman)?

Do you ever wish you were the opposite sex?

What would the advantages be?

Have you ever felt discriminated against because you are a man (woman)?

Have you ever had to do things you did not want to do because you are a man (woman)?

How important is sexual activity in your life?

Describe your current sexual outlet.

Are you satisfied with your sex life?

Are you dissatisfied with your partner's sexual functioning?

Is there anything about your (or your partner's) sexual activity (as individuals or as a couple) that you would like to change?

Do you have any questions or problems related to sex that you would like to discuss?

Do you fall in love at first sight?

Do you always fall in love with someone who reminds you of your parent of the opposite sex?

Can you easily accept the fact that your partner has loved others before you and not worry about how you compare with them?

How do you feel when your partner is not interested in sexual relations?

How do you feel after sexual relations?

What do you feel are the principal goals in sexual relations?

Do you feel a sense of rejection if a person you love tries to preserve his or her independence?

Can you accept your loved one's anger and still believe in his or her love?

Can you express your innermost thoughts and feelings to the person you love?

Modifications for the Older Adult

Has your desire for sex or interest in sex changed? If so, how?

Do you have problems with reaching orgasm or having discomfort during intercourse?

Do you have problems with obtaining or maintaining an erection or ejaculating?

Modifications for the Expectant Parent

How do you and your partner feel about breastfeeding your infant?

How do you feel when you see a woman nursing a child?

Which of these phrases best describes your concept of a pregnant woman: a person who will give birth to another person, a woman heavy with child, a woman bearing her husband's child, a mother-to-be?

How does being pregnant affect your sexual interest, desire, and functioning?

Does sexual activity during pregnancy affect the baby?

Should sexual activity be restricted by or during pregnancy or after pregnancy, and for what reasons?

Modifications for the Newborn

How do you and your partner feel when the baby touches its genitals?

What color do you usually choose in dressing your baby? Why?

Modifications for the Infant/Child/Adolescent

Is your family comfortable with household nudity?

What do you expect from the boys and girls in your family?

What do you remember about your childhood sex play?

Do you have a best friend?

What was the first sex information you received? (Consider parents, other sources.)

What information were you given? (Comfortable with it, information you needed?)

How do you feel about the changes taking place in your body? (Consider good, curious, anxious, enticing to others, sexy, vulnerable, awkward, pleased, secretive, proud, dirty, relieved, scared.)

Are you pleased with your body? (Consider comparison with others, want to make changes, attractive to others.)

What factors have been important in your decision to become or not become sexually active? (Consider peer pressure, partner pressure, family teachings, personal convictions, religious views, fear of pregnancy.)

Did you ever get a girl pregnant, or were you ever pregnant? (Consider outcome, feelings.)

What do you think about using contraceptives?

How do you feel about being sexually active?

How do you feel about your partner?

When and under what circumstances did you first experience feelings of love or being in love? (Consider length of relationship, feelings.)

When did you first experience kissing, holding, or touching?

When and under what circumstances did you first experience sexual arousal? (Consider feelings.)

How did you feel about these experiences?

Do you recall ever being unsure of your preference for gender of sexual partners?

How do you feel about this?

When did you first become interested in becoming sexually active?

Are your peers experimenting with sexual activity? (Consider adolescent.)

What do you think about this activity?

Can you remember the first time you were aware of being a boy or a girl? (Consider occasion, feelings.)

How do your parents feel about your friend, boyfriend or girlfriend?

In what ways do your beliefs and attitudes about dating and sex differ from those of your parents?

BIBLIOGRAPHY

Berliner, H. Sexuality assessments enhance quality of life. *N.J. Nurse,* 1986, *16*(4), 6–7.

Broderick, C. B., & Bernard, J. (Eds.). *The individual, sex and society.* Baltimore: Johns Hopkins University Press, 1969.

Butler, R. N., & Lewis, M. I. *Love and sex after sixty.* New York: Harper & Row, 1976.

Colman, A. D., & Colman, L. L. *Pregnancy: The psychological experience.* New York: Herder, 1971.

Cox, S., Doyle, K., Kammermann, S., & Valois, R. *Wellness rsvp.* Menlo Park, Calif.: Benjamin/Cummings, 1981.

Donlou, J. N. Psychosocial aspects of AIDS and AIDS related complex: A pilot study. *Journal of Psychosocial Oncology,* 1985, *3*(2), 39–55.

Ebersole, P., & Hess, P. *Toward healthy aging.* St. Louis: Mosby, 1981.

Elmassian, B., & Wilson, R. Assessment and diagnosis of sexual problems. *Nurse Practitioner*, 1982, *7*, 13–22.
Guarda, N., & Peterson, J. Screening for H.I.V. Antibodies. *Nursing 86*, 1986, 28–29.
Hill, P. M., & Humphrey, P. (Eds.). *Human growth and development throughout life: A nursing perspective*. New York: Wiley, 1982.
Hogan, R. M. *Human sexuality: A nursing perspective*. Norwalk, Conn.: Appleton-Century-Crofts, 1985.
Lion, E. M. Sexuality and adulthood. In E. M. Lion (Ed.), *Human sexuality in nursing process*. New York: Wiley, 1982.
Malasonos, L., Barkauskas, V., Moss, M., & Stoltenberg, A. *Health assessment*. St. Louis: Mosby, 1981.
Miles, L. *Sleep questionnaire and assessment of wakefulness*. Stanford, Calif.: Stanford University Medical Center, n.d.
Mims, F. H., & Swenson, M. *Sexuality: A nursing perspective*. New York: McGraw-Hill, 1980.
Sullivan, H. S. *The interpersonal theory of psychiatry*. New York: Norton, 1953.
Woods, N. F. *Human sexuality in health and illness*. St. Louis: Mosby, 1979.

UNIT 12

Medications

INTRODUCTION

Our society is bombarded by the media with information about various medications, over-the-counter drugs, and remedies. Local supermarkets, drugstores, and health-food facilities have counters lined with an overwhelming selection of powders, pills, capsules, liquids, and ointments to cure real and imagined ills. There are pills for sleeping and others to make one more alert. There are vitamins to make one healthy and medications to relieve constipation, diarrhea, "excess stomach acid," and common cold symptoms. Frequently one's choice of a remedy is influenced more by effective advertising than by knowledge about the suitability of the product in relationship to the problem.

Medication use is also influenced by beliefs and values learned by the person within the context of the family and culture. When a family member is ill, the sick roles and rituals are frequently distinctly defined within the family unit. For example, a care giver may suggest the person go to his room, put on pajamas, and get into bed. The care giver may then prepare the remedies perceived as appropriate to treat the sick individual. Care and remedies may include taking a temperature, giving some aspirin, offering hot tea with lemon and honey, or rubbing the chest with a menthol-based salve. Health-care professionals need to respect health-care practices within the various cultures in our society. After assessing the effectiveness of home remedies, appropriate aspects should be incorporated into the plan of care.

There are those who believe that if one pill is good, two are better. An example of this is the megavitamin use that is prevalent in our society today. Others believe that the use of little or no medication is the best solution. Some people will discontinue taking antibiotics when they begin to feel better, rather than taking the prescribed amount. One needs to evaluate the beliefs, values, and attitudes of the client toward medications. In addition, one needs to understand behaviors associated with self-medication and prescription use, as a part of the psychosocial assessment.

ADULT

Assessment of the adult's knowledge about medications and their use is important because the adult is not only responsible for self-medication but is often responsible for providing medications to children and other family members. When an adult is taking or giving medications, either over-the-counter or prescribed, it is important to determine the client's awareness of the name, action, dose, side effects, and precautions for each drug. Possession of this knowledge will enable the client to take and give drugs correctly. In addition to the effects of culture and persuasion, advertising, advice of friends and physician, or nurse recommendations may provide the basis for the decision to use a medication. Determining how the adult makes decisions as to the use of medications is a necessary step in the assessment process.

OLDER ADULT

Elderly persons consume a disproportionate share of the drugs and medications purchased in this country each year. This includes both prescription and over-the-counter preparations. This drug consumption by the elderly creates many overt problems and some that are not so apparent. Many elderly persons present for treatment in the health-care system as a result of drug reactions, interactions, or overmedication. Older persons who are institutionalized for confusional states often improve when some of their medications are withdrawn.

Because the elderly take so many medications and frequently take them incorrectly or inappropriately, functions within the psychosocial sphere of their lives are often affected. For example, misunderstanding about which pill is the diuretic and taking it at 5 PM rather than 9 AM may cause nocturia and thus disrupt sleep, resulting in the complaint of fatigue or lethargy on the following day.

Perhaps the most abused drugs among elderly persons are those in the laxative and stool-softener group. Many old people are constipated because of dietary changes or inactivity. There are many more, however, who think that they are constipated, perhaps because of the idea of previous generations that one must have a bowel movement each day. Many older people have no idea what a normal pattern of bowel movements for them would be because they have used laxatives, stool softeners, and even enemas daily for years.

The child-proof cap is a common problem for older persons as is the new tamper-proof packaging. Commonly these medications are taken for arthritis or other painful conditions and simply opening these containers can be a painful and frustrating experience as the bones and joints in hands and arms must work together to twist off the cap. Also, with decreased vision, the elderly person cannot see which way the arrow points, indicating which direction to turn the cap for removal. A simple solution to some of these problems is to ask the pharmacist not to use the child-proof containers, particularly when there are no small children in the home.

Most older persons take several drugs for different purposes. Often these have been prescribed by more than one health-care provider, each of whom may be unaware of the other prescriptions. Add to this the self-prescribing of over-the-counter medication or taking medications borrowed from friends or relatives, and the potential for untoward reactions is substantial.

EXPECTANT PARENT

Any female who is contemplating a pregnancy should curtail all medication use at least two months prior to becoming pregnant. During the beginning growth and development of the embryo, the mother does not even know she is pregnant, and the medications she is taking may indeed affect the neurological system of the baby.

Any medication taken by an expectant woman may adversely affect the developing embryo and fetus. The placenta does protect the fetus from some agents, but it is not an absolute barrier. The overall rule should be that the pregnant woman take no drugs during pregnancy. When any medication is administered during pregnancy, the benefits of the medication should outweigh any risks in its use. The mother needs to make an informed decision about what drugs she wishes to take after a discussion with her health-care provider.

NEWBORN

The newborn is usually healthy during the first 28 days of life and no medications are usually prescribed. If the mother is breast-feeding, prescription and self-medications will pass in the breast milk to the infant. Therefore, the influence of the medications taken by the breast-feeding mother on the newborn needs to be included as part of the assessment. An assessment of what a mother does for a cranky baby should also be included because some mothers may give a medication such as aspirin to comfort the baby.

INFANT/CHILD/ADOLESCENT

The main concept to be considered when assessing the young client is safety. Medications need to be kept in a safe place, such as a locked cabinet or one that has an alarm that will sound when the child tries to open it. Children need to be taught that medications are not candy but are taken for a distinct purpose. It is during the school-age and adolescent years that taking care of oneself develops. This process begins to instill a sense of responsibility in the young person. This sense of responsibility means that the child is now able to begin making some decisions about taking medications. The parent needs to allow the young person to begin to make decisions about the products to use and help him or her make wise choices about which ones not to use. Helping the young person in this decision-making process facilitates appropriate maturation and sets the stage for wise choices regarding medications as an adult.

QUESTIONNAIRE

ADULT

What are your feelings about taking drugs or medications?

Do you use precription drugs, over-the-counter drugs? (Consider taken regularly or irregularly, folk medicine [made from roots or leaves].)

Of the medications you are currently taking, how often taken, by what route (oral, ointment on skin, inhaled, etc.), and for what purpose?

Do you know what side effects are possible from your medicines?

Do you know when to take the medication to make it most effective and how the medication works? (Consider with milk, juice, meals, before or after meals.)

What do you do if a dose is missed?

What other medications have you taken in the past year?

What do you do with the remaining doses of medications no longer taken? (Consider how long retained, under what circumstances they would be used again.)

Where do you keep medications? (Consider safely away from children, labeled correctly, plainly.)

Are you allergic to any drugs? (Consider unpleasant reactions, drug type.)

What happened?

Where do you obtain your medications? (Consider cost, could generic drugs be substituted.)

Do you take a drug for the prescribed amount of time, avoid stretching to make it last longer, borrow or lend medicines?

Do you tell the physician all medicines you are taking whether or not prescribed by him or her?

Do you take more than prescribed, thinking that if one dose is helpful, two would be even better?

Do you avoid mixing alcohol with drugs? (Consider tranquilizers, barbiturates, antihistamines.)

Modifications for the Older Adult

Do you take more medication now than when you were younger?

Does this present any problems to you?

How do you remember to take your medications?

How do you avoid duplication in doses?

Do you have problems taking your medications? (Consider difficulty breaking tablets, giving self eye drops, opening child-proof containers, vision problems.)

Modifications for the Expectant Parent

How do you feel about taking medications while you are pregnant? (Consider decision-making process, effect on baby.)

Modifications for the Newborn

If breast-feeding, how do the medications you take affect your baby?

How is your baby comforted when not feeling well?

Modifications for the Infant/Child/Adolescent

Does your child know the difference between medication and candy?

What special things do you do to get your child to take medications?

What have you discussed with your child regarding use of medications?

How do you decide when and which over-the-counter medication to use? (Consider adolescent.)

BIBLIOGRAPHY

Bell, S. Guidelines for taking a complete drug history. *Nursing 80*, 1980, *10*, 10–11.

Cox, S., Doyle, K., Kammermann, S., & Valois, R. *Wellness rsvp*. Menlo Park, Calif.: Benjamin/Cummings, 1981.

Hurd, P. D., & Butkovich, S. L. Compliance problems and the older patient: Assessing functional . . . drug therapy. *Drug Intelligence and Clinical Pharmacy*, 1986, *20*(3), 228–231.

Ryan, P., & Falco, S. M. A pilot study to validate the etiologies and defining characteristics of the nursing diagnosis of noncompliance. *Nursing Clinics of North America,* 1985, *20*(4), 685–695.
Westfall, V. E. Methods for assessing compliance. *Topics in Clinical Nursing,* 1986, *7*(4), 23–30.
Yurick, A. G., Spier, B. E., Robb, S. S., Ebert, N. J. *The aged person and the nursing process,* 2nd ed. Norwalk, Conn.: Appleton-Century-Crofts, 1984.

UNIT 13

Substance Use

INTRODUCTION

Many people use a variety of substances in moderation throughout their life-span and do not experience any problems. On the other hand, millions of Americans have become dependent on some type of substance. Substance abuse is the taking into the body of any substance to the extent that it interferes recurringly in the functional life of the individual. The ingestion of any compound, such as drugs, alcohol, food, caffeine, or tobacco in amounts that are harmful to the individual's health and well-being constitutes substance abuse. Persons who are users usually are experiencing difficulties in several areas of life, encountering family, work, legal, health, and emotional problems.

How does an individual develop an addiction to any of these substances? When the client develops a problem or need that leads to tension and anxiety, some type of substance may be used to relieve those symptoms. If this behavior is frequently repeated, a psychological dependence occurs. The person who stops using the substance at this point will experience stress and anxiety, but no physical problems. The next part of the cycle is physical dependence, which usually follows the psychological dependence. At this point, the individual requires larger amounts of the substance to obtain the desired effect, and if the client stops using the substance a characteristic withdrawal syndrome will be manifested. As the individual tries to gain control of his or her life, this cycle may be stopped and started several times.

It is often difficult for health-care providers to identify and treat substance users. One of the first steps to be taken toward solution of this problem is for the nurse to analyze her or his feelings toward inappropriate substance use so as to be able to recognize how personal attitudes and feelings influence the ability to assess clients with this problem. To be effective in assisting this type of patient there must be a nonjudgmental attitude based on an understanding of self. Negative nonverbal behaviors on the part of the nurse will preclude assistance to the user.

ADULT

Adults are more likely than adolescents to use alcohol and prescription drugs rather than illegal substances. The pressures of starting a new career, having time for social activities, and starting a family may require long periods with less-than-adequate sleep. Stimulants such as caffeine, cocaine, or amphetamines may then be used by the young adult in an effort to remain alert enough to carry out daily activities. Tiring of this busy life-style, the adult who is trying to establish a career and deal with the problems of growing children may begin to take tranquilizers to cope with life stresses.

Our society accepts the use of some substances such as alcohol, tobacco, food, and drugs as a comfort measure. Therefore, the individual who begins to lose the ability to control the intake of these substances may not be recognized until the addiction has already developed. For this reason, it is important to assess each adult client for possible substance use.

OLDER ADULT

The older adult is less likely to use substances that have come to be known as "street drugs" and more likely to use or misuse prescriptions and over-the-counter preparations. Many older people are both overtly and covertly depressed. Untreated, these various levels of depression may lead to drug use as a means of coping with the depression. This use may range from the older woman who becomes dependent on tranquilizers to ward off the daily reminders of her unpleasant existence to the older man who succeeds in taking his own life by the use of drugs available to him.

A substantial number of persons among the elderly are thought to have varying degrees of dependence on drugs that have been prescribed over long periods of time in an effort to control chronic pain. If the client has taken the drug for some time, the value may be more psychological than physiological in relief of pain. Clearly this group of clients has some degree of drug dependence. Among health professionals the attitudes toward this dependence vary greatly. Some feel that no matter the age or circumstances of the client, assessing the client as drug-dependent requires that an effort be made to eliminate the problem. Others feel ambivalent. And still others believe that because the person is old, the drug has been taken for a long time, and it hasn't done any apparent harm, why worry about it?

In assessing substance use for the elderly person, factors such as short-term memory, chronic diseases present, state of mental health, living arrangements, activities, access to health care, and income must all be taken into consideration in arriving at an accurate assessment and an appropriate plan.

EXPECTANT PARENT

The unborn child is directly affected by the mother's substance use or abuse. Expectant mothers who smoke cigarettes place the fetus at high risk to suffer congenital anomalies and developmental disabilities. It is commonly found that babies born to mothers who smoke have lower birth weight, are smaller, and have diminished intellectual function. There is now a correlation between smoking in the home and sudden infant death syndrome.

Malformations also have been associated with maternal alcohol abuse. Undesirable results for the fetus that are linked to chronic alcohol exposure in utero include serious limitations in growth and mental and motor performance. The exact amount of alcohol that produces fetal alcohol syndrome has not been identified and is under investigation, along with the exact mechanisms by which this damage occurs to the fetus.

Narcotic addiction and drug abuse in women of child-bearing age are steadily increasing in the United States. A recent study conducted in seven major United States cities estimated between 4500 and 5000 newborns are born addicted to narcotics every year. Neonatal mortality for addicted newborns is six to eight times higher than that of nonaddicted newborns (Bobak & Jensen, 1984).

Zelson found that withdrawal symptoms were observed in 80 to 90 percent of infants born to narcotic-addicted women. There is currently no way to predict the severity of withdrawal or its onset. While there may be many physical complications for the expectant mother and unborn child, the psychosocial assessment must address the level of care and concern the expectant mother feels toward the fetus (Zelson, 1975).

NEWBORN

The mother–infant attachment process may be delayed or problematical in the case of addictions. The mother may need help to learn comfort methods for her baby. Swaddling, small feedings, cuddling, and rocking may need to be taught. Because of the mother's life-style, the baby may be a source of guilt to her. The child may be viewed as a burden who will interfere with her life-style of drug dependency. The mother may need counseling to promote a better self-concept and improve self-esteem. She will also need follow-up by community resources so that the health and well-being of the baby can be assured.

INFANT/CHILD/ADOLESCENT

Unfortunately, there is a trend in this country toward the use of drugs, alcohol, and tobacco by children of the grade-school age. Nurses and parents each have an important role in attempting to stem this alarming occurrence. The school nurse can be instrumental in preventing this problem by starting educational programs on substance use in the grade schools. Parents can prevent the problem by acting as role models rather than using such substances as alcohol and prescription drugs and then telling their children not to smoke marijuana.

Adolescence is a very intense period of growing and maturing. The intensity of this period and the discomfort associated with psychological growth may lead the adolescent to seek relief through experimentation with new behaviors. Also, the teenager is easily influenced by peers and current fads. Eager to test his or her capabilities and often dissatisfied with the adult world, the teenager may be motivated to experiment with drugs and other substances. It is easy to see how the addictive cycle could be reinforced during these vulnerable years.

QUESTIONNAIRE

ADULT

Do you consider overeating, alcohol intake, smoking tobacco, or drug use to be a serious personal problem for you?

Do you feel as though you are dependent on coffee, tea, soft drinks, alcohol, or any drug?

Do you believe that any of the medicines or drugs you have taken or are taking now are bad for your health?

Have you ever taken medicines or drugs to help you fall asleep, perk up, or control appetite?

Have you ever taken drugs or medicines for depression or other mental health problems?

Do you ever share your medication with someone or take drugs prescribed for others?

Do you consider yourself to be overweight?

Do you consider yourself to be a big, average, or small eater?

Where and with whom do you generally eat meals?

What foods do you like and dislike most?

Do you eat only at a designated place and/or time?

Is there any difficulty with eating?

What beverages do you drink each day? (Consider coffee, tea, cola, amount of each.)

Do you eat excessively? (Consider when bored, depressed, suffering from insomnia.)

Do you eat foods you know are not good for you?

Do you prefer eating alone, feel conspicuous or embarrassed when eating with others?

Do you sneak, hide food, eat, and drink in secrecy?

Do you feel self-conscious about how your body looks?

Do you gulp food or stuff yourself?

Do you crave sweets or indulge in them?

Do you eat on the run?

Do you eat when not hungry, have uncontrollable hunger urges, eating binges, meals or snacks after 7 PM, or eat within one hour of retiring?

Do you have feelings of anger, hostility, fatigue or feel as though you are in the midst of a "struggle"? (Consider diet, other abuses.)

Do certain people, problems, or situations trigger eating? (Consider who are they, why.)

How do you handle these situations?

Do you mix eating with other activities? (Consider reading, studying, watching TV.)

Do you eat slowly?

Do you use small dishes to make portions seem larger?

Do you avoid shopping when hungry?

Do you bake, broil, or steam foods to decrease caloric content?

Do you drink nonfat milk, cut down on foods that are high in sugar, keep problem foods out of the house, and use low-calorie food items for snacks?

Do you attempt to limit caloric intake when eating out?

Have you ever tried special diets? (Consider Weight Watchers, other methods to control your weight.)

Have you ever been placed on a special diet by a health-care provider for weight control?

For how long did you attempt these efforts and what was the outcome?

Do you smoke?

How much do you smoke in a 24-hour period? (Consider packs of cigarettes, number of cigars, pipe.)

Do you use any form of tobacco or tobacco substitute? (Consider snuff, chewing tobacco, nicotine gum, smokeless cigarette.)

When do you smoke or use tobacco?

Have you tried to stop? (Consider successful, reason for lack of success.)

Do you still want to quit?

Have you quit smoking or using tobacco products? (Consider how long ago, the amount used prior to stopping.)

Do you think cigarette smoking or other tobacco use is harmful to your health? (Consider damaging to your person, property, making you feel dependent, a messy habit.)

Is smoking hard for you to control?

Do you worry about the example you set for others?

Do you smoke or use tobacco products to perk yourself up, for pleasure or relaxation, when you are uncomfortable or upset about something?

Do you reach for a cigarette or tobacco source automatically?

Do you enjoy handling a cigarette?

Do you drink alcoholic beverages of any kind and how often?

How many drinks do you have in a 24-hour period? (Consider bottle/cans of beer, glasses of wine, shots of liquor.)

At what time of day do you drink?

Are you preoccupied with thoughts of alcohol?

Do you usually drink alone or when others are not drinking?

Do you worry about protecting your supply so you won't run out?

Do you drink more when under stress?

Do you drink more than planned or become intoxicated, and how often?

Does it take increasing amounts of alcohol to feel the effect?

Do you have lapses of memory, blackouts, hallucinations, shakes or DTs?

Have you ever injured yourself or others while drinking?

Has your drinking ever caused you to be ill or hospitalized?

Have you ever been in jail or arrested because of drinking?

Has your alcohol consumption ever caused any family or employment problems?

Do you or your family ever worry about your drinking?

Have you tried to stop drinking; were you successful?

Do other family members drink alcohol and how much?

Are there any problem drinkers in your family?

Does the cost of alcohol create any financial problems?

Have you ever attended any therapy sessions because you were concerned about your drinking behavior?

Do you consume significantly less alcohol at present than in the past?

What was the reason for change?

What medications do you take routinely? (Consider why, for how long.)

What medications do you take when needed and for what reasons?

Have you ever taken or used illegal substances? (Consider narcotics, cocaine, LSD, PCP, marijuana, peyote, stimulants, depressants, glue, or paint sniffing.)

How often and for how long did you use these drugs?

Have you used any drugs through your veins? If so, have you shared syringes and/or needles?

Does the possibility of AIDS concern you as a result of these experiences or others?

Have you ever been in trouble with the law for using or selling illegal drugs; what happened?

Have you ever taken any drug for "kicks"?

Have you ever been treated for drug overdose or other health problem related to drug use?

Modifications for the Older Adult

Do you have any concerns about taking medicines appropriately?

Has the way you use medications changed as you have aged?

Modifications for the Expectant Parent

Do you feel that the medicines or drugs you are now taking will hurt the baby?

What are some of the food or drug cravings you have had during this pregnancy?

Has the father of the baby experienced any food or drug cravings?

How do you feel about your weight gain during pregnancy?

How does this baby's father like your weight gain?

During this pregnancy have you placed yourself on a special diet to control your weight?

How do you feel about smoking, drinking, or drug use during your pregnancy?

How does the baby's father feel about smoking around you and the baby?

How do you think your smoking, drinking or drug use will affect your baby?

Modifications for the Newborn

How does your baby behave?

Do you smoke around your baby?

Modifications for the Infant/Child/Adolescent

Do you experiment with drugs?

What do your peers think about drug, alcohol and cigarette use?

Do any of your peers use drugs, alcohol or tobacco products?

Do you feel pressure from your friends to use these substances?

Do your parents use any of these substances?

Have you ever discussed the use of these substances with your parents?

With whom do you feel you can discuss this subject?

Do you have any classes at school to discuss these subjects?

What do you think about having discussions on these subjects?

REFERENCES

Bobak, I. M., & Jensen, M. D. *Essentials of maternity nursing*. St. Louis: Mosby, 1984, pp. 955–956.

Zelson, C. Acute management of neonatal addiction. *Addictive Diseases: An International Journal*, 1975, 2(1), 159–168.

BIBLIOGRAPHY

Alexander, L. L. Smoking and smoking cessation: Occupational health issue. *Journal of the American Association of Occupational Health Nursing,* 1986, *34*(8), 383–387.

Bryant, S. O. Psychiatric nursing assessment of the eating disorder client. *Topics in Clinical Nursing,* 1986, *8*(1), 57–66.

Burkhalter, P. K. *Nursing care of the alcoholic and drug abuser.* New York: McGraw-Hill, 1975.

Carr, G. S. AIDS and AIDS-related conditions: Screening for populations at risk. *Nurse Practitioner,* 1986, *11*(10), 25–26, 29, 32–34.

Cox, S., Doyle, K., Kammerman, S., & Valois, R. *Wellness rsvp.* Menlo Park, Calif.: Benjamin/Cummings, 1981.

Crawshaw, J. P. Anorexia and bulimia: The earliest clues. *Patient Care,* 1985, *19*(18), 80–83, 86–90, 93–95.

Durell, J., & Bukoski, W. Preventing substance abuse: The state of the art. *Public Health Reports,* 1984, *99*(1), 23–31.

Ellor, J. R., & Kurz, D. J. Misuse and abuse of prescription and nonprescription drugs by the elderly. *Nursing Clinics of North America,* 1982, *17*(2), 319–330.

Estes, N. J., & Heinmann, M. E. *Alcoholism: Development, consequences and interventions.* St. Louis: Mosby, 1982.

Francis, G., & Munjas, B. *Manual of socialpsychologic assessment.* New York: Appleton-Century-Crofts, 1976.

The frightening statistics on infant addiction. *Parade,* November 18, 1984, p. 9.

Keen, S. *The pure, the impure and the paranoid.* New York: Ziff-Davis, 1976.

McArdle, K., & Duphorne, P. Addictive behavior. In S. Lewis & I. Collier (Eds.), *Medical–surgical nursing: Assessment and management of clinical problems.* New York: McGraw-Hill, 1982.

National Institutes of Health, Public Health Service. *Why do you smoke?* U.S. Department of Health, Education and Welfare Publication No. 80-1822-A. Washington, D.C.: U.S. Government Printing Office, 1980.

Niven, R. G. Adolescent drug abuse. *Hospital and Community Psychiatry,* 1986, *37*(6), 596–607.

Ogur, B. Long day's journey into night: Women and prescription drug abuse. *Women and Health,* 1986, *11*(1), 99–115.

Pallikkathayil, L., & Tweed, S. Substance abuse: Alcohol and drugs during adolescence. *Nursing Clinics of North America,* 1983, *18*(2), 313–321.

Pritchard, J. A., MacDonald, P. C., & Grant, N. F. *Williams Obstetrics,* 17th ed. Norwalk, Conn.: Appleton-Century-Crofts, 1985.

Savage, T. V. Investigating the social aspects of alcohol use. *Health Education,* 1984, *15*(1), 49–50.

Selzer, M., Vinokur, A., & Van Roojen, L. A self-administered short Michigan alcoholism screening test (SMAST [Short Michigan Alcoholism Screening Test]). *Journal on Studies of Alcohol*, 1975, *36*(1), 117–126.
Stephenson, J. N., Mobero, P., Daniels, B. J., & Robertson, J. F. Treating the intoxicated adolescent. A need for comprehensive services. *Journal of the American Medical Association*, 1984, *251*, 1884.
Whaley, L., & Wong, D. *Nursing care of infants and children*. St. Louis: Mosby, 1983.

INDEX